ANTIBODIES

VOLUME 2: NOVEL TECHNOLOGIES AND THERAPEUTIC USE

ANTIBODIES

VOLUME 2: NOVEL TECHNOLOGIES AND THERAPEUTIC USE

Edited by

G. Subramanian
Littlebourne, Kent, United Kingdom

Springer Science+Business Media, LLC

Library of Congress Cataloging-in-Publication Data

Antibodies / edited by G. Subramanian.
    p. ; cm.
    Includes bibliographical references and index.
    Contents: v. 1. Production and purification -- v. 2. Novel technologies and therapeutic use.
    ISBN 0-306-48245-2 (v. 1) -- ISBN 0-306-48315-7 (v. 2) -- ISBN 0-306-48334-3
    (divisible set)
        1. Monoclonal antibodies--Synthesis. 2. Monoclonal antibodies--Therapeutic use. 3.
    Monoclonal antibodies--Biotechnology. I. Subramanian, G., 1935-
        [DNLM: 1. Antibodies, Monoclonal--isolation & purification. 2. Antibodies,
    Monoclonal--therapeutic use. 3. Biotechnology--methods. 4. Chromatography--methods.
    QW 575.5.A6 A6283 2004]
    TP248.65.M65A55 2004
    615'.37--dc22
                                                                            2003069160

ISBN 978-1-4613-4702-6   ISBN 978-1-4419-8877-5 (eBook)
DOI 10.1007/978-1-4419-8877-5

©2004 Springer Science+Business Media Dordrecht
Originally published by Kluwer Academic Publishers/Plenum Publishers, New York in 2004
Softcover reprint of the hardcover 1st edition
http://www.wkap.nl/

10 9 8 7 6 5 4 3 2 1

A C.I.P. record for this book is available from the Library of Congress

Permissions for books published in Europe: permissions@wkap.nl
Permissions for books published in the United States of America: permissions@wkap.com

Preface

It is now over one hundred years since von Behring and Kitsato first concluded experiments that led to the use of passive immunisation, employing antibodies raised in animals against tetanus and diphtheria toxins. The advancement of technology both in manufacturing purity product in a cost effective way and the clinical research has proved that antibodies are one of the most successful products in biotechnology.

Monoclonal antibodies account for between one-third and one-half of all pharmaceutical products in development and human clinical trials. Both the nature of monoclonal antibody therapies and the relatively large size of the monoclonal antibody dictate the production requirements, for many of these therapeutics the monoclonal antibody product will be 100 kilogrammes or more per year. It is widely acknowledged that there is currently a worldwide shortage of biomanufacturing capacity, and the active pharmaceutical ingredient material requirements for these products are expected to increase. Thus the industry is looking for new sources and extensive studies are being carried out not only for alternative technology to meet the needs but also to reveal the new therapeutic applications of antibodies.

This book brings to the forefront current advances in novel technologies for the manufacturing of monoclonal antibodies and also their extensive clinical importance. The first four chapters give an overview of the new technologies and the successful application in the manufacture of monoclonal antibodies with clinical purity. The next chapters address the application of antibodies in cancer therapy and functional genomic therapy. The last chapter projects the importance of antibodies and the prospects of antibody engineering and therapy for the future.

It is my hope that this book will bring together accumulated knowledge in a way which will promote the advancement of the antibody field, which will continue to grow and develop new antibodies that are useful to society at large.

I gratefully acknowledge the authors for their time and motivation in preparing their contributions, without which this book would not have been possible. I should be most grateful for any suggestions, which could serve to improve future editions of this book

Finally I would like to thank Jo Lawrence of Kluwer Academic/Plenum for her keen interest and help throughout the completion of this book.

G. Subramanian

Contributors

Jean-Pierre Abastado
Immuno Designed Molecule (IDM)
172 rue de Charonne
75011 Paris Cedex 11
France

Adrian Auf Der Maur
ESBATech AG
Wagistrasse 21
8952 Zürich-Schlieren
Switzerland

Fabrice Auzelle
Immuno Designed Molecule (IDM)
172 rue de Charonne
75011 Paris Cedex 11
France

David Azira
Department of Radiation Oncology
CRLC Val d'Aurelle-Paul Lamarque
F-34298 Montpellier Cedex 5
France

Alcide Barberis
ESBATech AG
Wagistrasse 21
8952 Zürich-Schlieren
Switzerland

Jacques Bartholeyns
Immuno Designed Molecule (IDM)
172 rue de Charonne
75011 Paris Cedex 11
France

Emmanuelle Bonnin
INSERM U255
Centre de Recherches Biomedicales des Cordeliers
15, rue de l'Ecole de Médicine
75270 Paris Cedex 06
France

Egisto Boschetti
Ciphergen Biosystems-Biosepra
48, Avenue des Genottes
F-95800, Cergy
France

Aurélie Boyer
Immuno Designed Molecule (IDM)
172 rue de Charonne
75011 Paris Cedex 11
France

Manuela Campiglio
Molecular Targeting Unit
Department of Experimental Oncology
Isituto Nazionale Tumori
Milan
Italy

Gabrielle Caravelho
INSERM U542
Paris-Sud University
101 rue de Tolbiac
7654 Paris Cedex 13
France

Alain Chapel
Institute of Radioprotection and Nuclear Safety
IRSN/DAHD/SARAM
Fontenay–aux–Roses
France

Olivier Deas
INSERM U542
Paris-Sud University
101 rue de Tolbiac
75654 Paris Cedex 13
France

X. K. Deng
Meridian Bioscience
3471 River Hills Drive
Cincinnati
OH 45244
USA

Dimiter S. Dimitrov
Laboratory of Experimental and Computational Biology
Center for Cancer Research
NCI-Frederick, NIH
Bldg 469, Room 246
P.O. Box B, Miller Drive
Frederick
MD 21702-1201
USA

Jean-Bernard Dubois
Department of Radiation Oncology
CRLC Val d'Aurelle-Paul Lamarque
F-34298 Montpellier Cedex 5
France

Antoine Dürrbach
INSERM U542
Paris-Sud University
Rue de Tolbiac
75654 Paris Cedex 13
France

Christian Frisch
MorphoSys AG
Lena-Christ-Strasse 48
D-82152 Martinsried/Planegg
Germany

Francois Hirsch
INSERM U542
Paris-Sud University
101 rue de Tolbiac
75654 Paris Cedex 13
France

Sylvie Jacod
Immuno Designed Molecule (IDM)
172 rue de Charonne
75011 Paris Cedex 11
France

Christel Larbouret
Immunociblago des Tumeurs et Ingenierie des Anticorps
EMI-0227 INSERM, Université Montpellier 1
CRLC Val d'Aurelle-Paul Lamarque
F-34298 Montpellier Cedex 5
France

Peter Lichtlen
ESBATech AG
Wagistrasse 21
8952 Zürich-Schlieren
Switzerland

Delphine Loirat
Immuno Designed Molecule (IDM)
172 rue de Charonne
75011 Paris Cedex 11
France

Andrès McAllister
Immuno Designed Molecule (IDM)
172 rue de Charonne
75011 Paris Cedex 11
France

Sylvie Ménard
Molecular Targeting Unit
Department of Experimental Oncology
Isituto Nazionale Tumori
Milan
Italy

K. John Morrow Jr.
Meridian Bioscience
3471 River Hills Drive
Cincinnati
OH 45244
USA

Maxime Moulard
BioCytex
140 Chemin de l'Armee d'Afrique
13010 Marseille
France

Ralf Ostendorp
MorphoSys AG
Lena-Christ-Strasse 48
D-82152 Martinsried/Planegg
Germany

Mahmut Ozashin
Department of Radiation Oncology
Centre Hospitalier Universitaire Vaudois
CH 1011 Lausanne
Switzerland

André Pèlegrin
Immunociblago des Tumeurs et Ingenierie des Anticorps
EMI-0227 INSERM, Université Montpellier 1
CRLC Val d'Aurelle-Paul Lamarque
F-34298 Montpellier Cedex 5
France

Serenella M. Pupa
Molecular Targeting Unit
Department of Experimental Oncology
Isituto Nazionale Tumori
Milan
Italy

Didier Prigent
Immuno Designed Molecule (IDM)
172 rue de Charonne
75011 Paris Cedex 11
France

T. Shantha Raju
CarboWorld
1010 Hadden Drive
San Mateo
CA 94402
USA

Bruno Robert
Immunociblago des Tumeurs et Ingenierie des Anticorps
EMI-0227 INSERM, Université Montpellier 1
CRLC Val d'Aurelle-Paul Lamarque
F-34298 Montpellier Cedex 5
France

Steve Sensoli
Biotechnology Consultant
9000 Joy Road
Plymouth
MI 481780
USA

Sophie Siberil
INSERM U255
Centre de Recherches Biomedicales des Cordeliers
15, rue de l'Ecole de Médicine
75270 Paris Cedex 06
France

Elda Tagliabue
Molecular Targeting Unit
Department of Experimental Oncology
Isituto Nazionale Tumori
Milan
Italy

Jean-Luc Teillaud
INSERM U255
Centre de Recherches Biomedicales des Cordeliers
15, rue de l'Ecole de Médicine
75270 Paris Cedex 06
France

Kathrin Tissot
ESBATech AG

Wagistrasse 21
8952 Zürich-Schlieren
Switzerland

Dominique Thierry
Institute of Radioprotection and Nuclear Safety
IRSN/DAHD/SARAM
Fontenay-aux-Roses
France

Margit Urban
MorphoSys AG
Lena-Christ-Strasse 48
D-82152 Martinsried/Planegg
Germany

Mei-Yun Zhang
BRP, SAIC-Frederick Inc.
Bldg 469, Room 131
P.O. Box B, Miller Drive
Frederick
MD 21702-1202
USA

Contents

Chapter 1

TRANSGENIC TECHNOLOGY FOR MONOCLONAL ANTIBODY PRODUCTION
An overview of transgenic animal and plant systems

Steve Sensoli
Biotechnology consultant from Ann Arbor, MI, USA, formerly with GeneWorks, Inc.

1. INTRODUCTION

Monoclonal antibodies account for between one-third and one-half of all pharmaceutical products in development and in human clinical trials. Both the nature of monoclonal antibody therapies, and the relatively large size of the monoclonal antibody molecules dictate that the production requirements for many of these therapeutic monoclonal antibody products will be 100 kilograms or more per year. It is widely acknowledged that there is currently a worldwide shortage of biomanufacturing capacity, and that the gap between biomanufacturing capacity and the active pharmaceutical ingredient material requirements for these products is expected to increase.

Transgenics is one possible way to alleviate this biomanufacturing capacity shortfall with relatively inexpensive, large-scale production of recombinant proteins. Transgenic avians, mammals and plants have all proven capable of producing monoclonal antibodies and other recombinant proteins.

An overview of these three groups of transgenic systems is presented to assist in the understanding, evaluation and comparison of the various transgenic methods available.

Antibodies, Volume 2: Novel Technologies and Therapeutic Use
Edited by G. Subramanian, Kluwer Academic/Plenum Publishers, New York 2004

1

2.   THE GROWING NEED FOR LARGE-SCALE BIOMANUFACTURING SYSTEMS

Between 1982 and 2002 there were 235 therapeutic biopharmaceutical medicines and vaccines (including approvals for new indications) approved for use in humans, more than half of those were approved in the last five years alone. The growing demand for these products and the development of additional recombinant protein-based therapeutics has created a well-documented shortfall in the worldwide biomanufacturing capacity. Products must now compete for bioreactor space, with some approved products being manufactured in short supply. To complicate matters further, hundreds of additional products that will require biomanufacturing are currently in development. Approximately one-third to one-half of those products in development are monoclonal antibodies (MAbs).

MAbs require a great deal of manufacturing capacity. The majority of small-molecule pharmaceutical products are used in relatively small doses – typically in the milligram to hundred milligram range. MAbs, on the other hand, require much larger doses – up to several grams of Active Pharmaceutical Ingredient (API) per patient. There are several reasons for this disparity. First, therapeutic MAbs are used to block cell receptor sites and the active sites of other proteins in the body. In order to act quickly and effectively, a large excess of the MAb molecules are required to seek out and block all of the targeted sites. Second, MAbs are significantly larger molecules than the majority of small molecule APIs. Additionally, the nature of many of the conditions and diseases to be treated by MAbs will likely require a regimen of doses.

The shortage of biomanufacturing capacity has been the cause for at least one notable (and highly profitable) biopharmaceutical product that could not be manufactured in great enough quantity to meet the market demand. There are estimates of several hundred million dollars in lost revenues for this one product alone. Worse than lost revenues, however, is the great deal of bad will garnered by any company whose product is backordered. In such cases, it is not uncommon to use an unbiased (yet trivial) lottery method to determine which patients will receive the critical and/or potential lifesaving product.

One might expect that many other biopharmaceutical products were also manufactured in short supply and that many other promising products were not even introduced since they could not be manufactured in production-scale quantities.

One reason for the shortage of biomanufacturing capacity is that production-scale bioreactors take 3-5 years to construct, qualify, produce validation lots and adequately train the equipment operators. Additionally, these bioreactors are expensive, often costing $75-$100 million or more for the production capabilities portion alone, and not including the downstream processing areas that typically accompany the bioreactors. The decision to make such a substantial capital commitment is a tough enough, but the decision to construct the facility must often be made years in advance of knowing whether the product that the facility is designed to produce will actually be approved by the regulatory agencies.

If there is not enough biomanufacturing capacity for the therapeutic products that already have regulatory approval, how will we produce enough API to fulfil the requirements for all of the new MAb and other recombinant protein-based products being developed? Some people believe that transgenics will provide a safe and inexpensive biomanufacturing platform with nearly limitless capacity constraints.

3. TRANSGENIC SYSTEMS

The word transgenics is a combination of *trans* (to transfer or change) and *genics* (relating to a gene or genome). It is the name for both a general field of science and for an industry. Transgenic technology involves the transfer of a gene or DNA sequence from one organism into the cells or genome of a genetically different type of organism. This transfer is usually accomplished by standard genetic engineering techniques, however cruder methods (*e.g.* gene guns) have been successfully employed in some transgenic systems.

This description of transgenics can pertain to a wide range of organisms developed for a variety of purposes, including basic research and improving the agronomic traits of plants (and animals) that are intended to enter the human food supply. Indeed, the process of transgenseis is accomplished in laboratories throughout the world. However, for the remainder of this chapter the word *transgenics* refers solely to transgenic animals and plants used in the production of recombinant biopharmaceutical MAbs and other therapeutic proteins.

As was mentioned above, the dosing regimen and molecular size of therapeutic Mabs is relatively large. Therefore, any biomanufacturing system used to produce them should have the capability of scaling up to a production level of 100kg or more per year.

For each of the transgenic systems discussed in this chapter, the capital costs and unit production costs are expected to be considerably less than those for the traditional bioreactor systems. To date, no therapeutic product derived from a transgenic animal or plant source has been approved by the appropriate regulatory agencies for use in humans. Therefore, no final costs for transgenics have been published. However, informal discussions with many of these companies indicate their transgenics facilities are projected to cost less than 10% of the cost of a bioreactor facility having comparable production capacity, and will require less than one year to construct. Likewise, the per-gram production costs of MAbs and other therapeutic proteins are also projected to be less than 10% of the cost of production in a bioreactor.

Within the realm of transgenics there are many species employed. Each of these species/systems is attractive because their harvest is bountiful and easily accomplished. The marketplace has organised these systems into three basic categories. They are, in alphabetical order:

1. Avians (primarily chickens) that produce the recombinant proteins in their egg white.

2. Mammals that produce the recombinant proteins in their milk or blood.

3. Plants that produce the recombinant proteins in the seeds, the fruit, the leaves, and elsewhere in the plant.

There are several methods of transgenesis used for each transgenic species, and many companies racing to be the industry leader for each of that system. The technological methodology employed by each of those companies is a function of their technological knowledge base, the species of animal used and the company's intellectual property position. The issues of technical expertise and intellectual property rights are even more acute in the case of MAb production since two genes (one coding for the heavy chain and one coding for the light chain) must not only be successfully transferred to the recipient organism, but they must also be expressed in close proximity to each other so that the chains "find" each other and become linked.

A brief description of each of the avain, mammalian and plant transgenic systems follows.

3.1   Avians

Chickens are the primary species used for production of recombinant proteins in the eggs of transgenic avians. Two commonly asked questions are "Why not use turkeys which have larger eggs than chickens, or ostriches which have even larger eggs?" and "Why not use quail which have a shorter generation time than chickens [so as to shorten the timelines for developing the flock's founding rooster and scale-up of the production flock]?". The answer to both of these questions is: over the past century, chicken egg production has been optimized by the food egg industry. The egg size, animal breeding programs and the equipment for housing the birds and collecting / processing the eggs have all been optimized for both high production volume and low production cost. This fact alone makes all other avian species far less efficient.

The Single Comb White Leghorn hen, the primary breed used for egg production in the United States, lays 250 eggs or more per year (Stadelman, 1995) each egg averages 60 grams in total mass (Li-Chan et al, 1995), about 3.6 grams of which are egg white proteins (Li-Chan et al, 1995, Sugino et al, 1997), for a total production of 900 grams of protein per bird, per year. If one can harness just a small percentage of this production capability for production of recombinant proteins, in can be envisioned that a 10,000 bird facility (which is quite small by egg-laying industry standards) could produce 100 kilograms of recombinant MAb per year.

There are several methods for generating transgenic avians, and each of the avian companies listed in this section uses one or more of the following technologies to make their transgenic animals.

1) Retroviruses. A retrovirus carrying the transgenes coding for the desired MAb can be used to infect the developing embryo with the goal of integrating the transgenes into the genome of the embryo's germ cells. This embryo then hatches as a chimeric, or partially transgenic G_0 bird. Not all of the germ cells are typically infected in this process, so only some the cells that go on to become the rooster's testes will have had the opportunity to integrate the transgenes. This means that usually only some of the sperm-producing cells in a chimeric rooster will produce sperm containing the transgenes and, therefore, the rooster's semen will be a mix of transgenic and non-transgenic sperm cells. Chicks resulting from insemination by the transgenic sperm will be fully transgenic hens and roosters (G_1). One more generation of animals is then sired by one of the G_1 "founder" roosters so that all of the offspring (G_2 G_3 G_4 ...) will carry the transgene. From G_2 on, the hens should lay eggs containing the recombinant protein coded for by the transgene, and the roosters can be used to propagate the flock.

2) Stem cell / primordial germ cell. This is the direct manipulation of embryonic stem cells (ESC) and/or primordial germ cells (PGCs). This method directly addresses the goal of retroviral infection of the embryo described in the above paragraph. Rather than infecting the entire embryo with the hope that the retrovirus carrying the transgene will find at least some of the PGCs and transfer the transgenes, direct manipulation of the PGCs should result in a greater rate of transgenesis. As with the retroviral method, transgenesis of all of the PGCs cannot be guaranteed because of the difficulty in locating the relatively few PGCs in an embryo of perhaps 50,000 cells. So the first generation of these chicks are also chimeric birds.

3) Sperm-Mediated Transgenesis (SMT). In SMT, a transgene is tranfected, infected, linked to, or otherwise transferred to the rooster sperm. The sperm with the transgene is then used to inseminate egg-laying hens. The offspring resulting from the sperm / transgene combination will be transgenic. One advantage of this method is that, since all of the cells in the first generation birds descended from a single transgenic cell, the first generation animals produced are fully transgenic G_1 birds. Compared to the retroviral and stem cell methods, one generation (six months for avians) is saved in the development time.

4) Pronuclear injection. In pronuclear injection, the transgene is linked to a promoter and any other required genetic sequences to form the expression cassette. This expression cassette is then injected into newly fertilized oocytes near the pronucleus and the oocytes are then inserted into surrogate hens. This method has not been well described in the literature, but may have a great degree of technical difficulty since there are multiple pronuclei on the yolk of each hen's egg. As with the SMT method, all of the cells in the first generation birds have descended from a single transgenic cell, so the first generation animals produced are fully transgenic G_1 birds.

Each of these methods of transgenesis have advantages and disadvantages relative to the others, and all of them are still being improved. The key development parameters that are evaluated include the degree of technical difficulty, the hatch rate, the rate of transgenesis and the size limitations for the transgene(s).

Table 1.1. List of Prominent Avian Transgenics Companies

Company name (location)
Avigenics (Athens, GA)
BioAgri (City of Industry, CA)
Cima Biotechnology/ACT (Worcester, MA)
GeneWorks (Ann Arbor, MI)
Origen Therapeutics (Burlingame, CA)
TransXenoGen (Shrewsbury, MA)
Viragen (Plantation, FL)
Vivalis (Nantes, France)

As of December 31, 2002

3.2   Mammals

The mammals most commonly used for production of recombinant antibodies and other proteins are cows, goats, sheep and rabbits. These animals can be engineered to produce recombinant MAbs in their milk. As with egg production in chickens, milk production has also been market optimized for production quantity and price – especially in cows and goats.

In deciding which mammal would be the best to use for production of a given recombinant protein, one must consider several factors including the quantity and timing of product needed, the eventual scale of product required, development and production costs, type of animal housing facilities available, and the development timeline.

Their primary methods of mammalian animal transgenesis include nuclear transfer and pronuclear injection.

1) Nuclear transfer. This process generally involves the fusing of a donor cell or its nucleous which has been engineered to contain the transgene, with an enucleated oocyte. First the donor cell is treated so as to have the transgene, a promoter sequence and other required genetic sequences incorporated. Then, an oocyte is isolated and enucleated. Finally, the donor cell and the enucleated oocyte are fused (by electroporation or by chemical means), and cultured for a short time. The newly engineered oocyte is then implanted into the womb of a surrogate mother.

2) Pronuclear injection. For pronuclear injection, the transgene is linked to a promoter and any other required genetic sequences to form the expression cassette. This expression cassette is then injected into newly fertilized oocytes near the pronucleus. As with nuclear transfer, the newly engineered oocyte is then implanted into the womb of a surrogate mother.

Both methods of mammalian transgesis produce some offspring that are fully transgenic since all of its cells will have descended from the engineered oocyte. The transgenic females produce the recombinant protein and the transgenic males are mated to expand the herd.

One of the companies listed below performs nuclear transfer of a Human Artificial Chromosome to engineer transgenic cattle embryos that are implanted into surrogate mothers. Some of the resulting offspring will produce human polyclonal antibodies in response to the introduction of an antigenic substance. While this process does not yield monoclonal antibodies, it is notable within the realm of mammalian transgenics.

Table 1.2. List of Prominent Mammalian Transgenics Companies

Company name (location)
BioProtein (Paris, France)
Gala Design (Sauk City, WI)
GTC Biotherapeutics (Framingham, MA)
Hematech (Sioux Falls, SD)
Nexia Biotechnologies (Montreal, Canada)
PPL Therapeutics (Edinburgh, UK)

As of December 31, 2002

3.3   Plants

Certainly the most diverse category of transgenic systems for the production of recombinant monoclonal antibodies is the plants. Many plants are being used for this purpose, however the most common plants are alfalfa, corn, *Lemna*, potato, rice, safflower, and tobacco. The recombinant protein may be produced in the leaves, stems, roots, seeds and even in the seed oil.

As with the transgenic avian and mammal systems, many of the techniques and equipment used for planting, cultivation, harvesting and storage of the transgenic crops are the same as those that have been used and optimized for food production. Therefore, most of the equipment required is readily available and inexpensive. These favourable economics may not, however, extend to the processes required for extraction and purification of the recombinant protein from transgenic plants.

There are basically two schemes used to generate a crop of transgenic plants. The first is to transform individual plant cells and allow them to grow up to full sized founder plants, expanding the crop both at the individual plant cell culture stage, and with standard growing and seed production methods similar to those employed in food agriculture. The second method is to transform growing and fully-grown plants.

Transforming individual plant cells can be accomplished with plant viral vectors or with a "gene gun".

The plant viral vector method is similar to the viral methods used for transforming avian and mammalian cells and embryos. The process starts by linking the gene coding for the desired protein to a promoter and any other required genetic sequences (including an antibiotic-resistance gene for selection) to produce an expression cassette. This cassette is then delivered into plant cells using plant viruses. The plant cells are selected by antibiotics, expanded in culture, then allowed to grow to full size.

In the gene gun process, the transgene cassette is coated onto micro particles such as gold or tungsten. These coated particles are then "fired" at plant cells with blasts of compressed air. The particles penetrate the plant cells, releasing some of the expression cassettes which then diffuse into the nucleus and integrate into the cells' genome. The plant cells are selected by antibiotics, expanded in culture, then allowed to grow to full size.

Portions of adult plants can also be transformed using viral vectors and gene guns. A solution of the viral vectors carrying the expression cassette is sprayed or rubbed onto the plants where it can be taken up by the plant cells. The expression cassette can also be introduced into the cells of adult plants using a gene gun. The cells that take up the virus by either method described will progress as above, except that the transformed plants are not usually selected for antibiotic resistance. Some of the plant's cells will express the gene.

Since the plants involved are such a diverse group, the expression levels in plants are best compared in units of kilograms of recombinant protein per acre of transgenic crop. In public presentations, several of the companies listed in Table 1.3 have reported between one and ten kilograms of recombinant protein per acre.

Table 1.3. List of Prominent Plant Transgenics Companies

Company name (location)	Primary plants used
AltaGen Bioscience (Morgan Hill, CA)	Potato
Biolex (Pittsboro, NC)	*Lemna*
Croptech (Blacksburg, VA)	Tobacco
Epicyte Pharmaceutical (San Diego, CA)	Corn, rice
Large Scale Biology (Vacaville, CA)	Tobacco
Medicago (Quebec City, Canada)	Alfalfa
Meristem Therapeutics (Clermont-Ferrand, France)	Corn, tobacco
Monsanto Protein Technologies (St. Louis, MO)	Corn
MPB Cologne (Cologne, Germany)	Potato
Planet Biotechnology (Hayward, CA)	Tobacco
ProdiGene (College Station, TX)	Corn
SemBioSys (Calgary, Canada)	Safflower

As of December 31, 2002

4.　　WHICH TRANSGENIC SYSTEM IS RIGHT FOR YOU?

Transgenics technology will be very useful for the large-scale biomanufacturing requirements of MAbs. But how does one decide which transgenic system to use? It is difficult to directly compare such diverse systems, but getting the answers to certain questions will help in the decision-making process. The characteristics of the MAb and the transgenic system employed must both be considered. Below is a non-exhaustive list of questions that can be helpful in determining which transgenic system (and which Contract Manufacturing Organization – CMO) is appropriate for the biomanufacturing of a given antibody.

4.1　　Monoclonal antibody-related questions

a) Is the MAb post-translationally modified?
b) What is the size of the gene construct that codes for the MAb (*i.e.* will the gene fit into the expression vector)?

c) Will the MAb injure or kill the host production animal or plant if it is expressed or released outside of the intended expression tissues?
d) What are the product development and marketing timelines?
e) What are the product development and marketing material requirements?

4.2   Technology-related questions

a) What is the method of transgenesis used?
b) Has the method of transgenesis been proven to stably integrate a transgene?
c) Can the method selected produce product under Good Manufacturing Practices (GMP) conditions?
d) From the date the CMO receives the DNA, how many months will it take to receive the first MAb sample?
e) From the date the CMO receives the DNA, how many months will it take to receive the first GMP-quality MAb?
f) Will the scaleup timeline match the product development timeline? That is, will the transgenic system be capable of supplying materials throughout the product development cycle?
g) Will the transgenic system be capable of scaling up to meet the projected peak sales?
h) What is the expected average annual output (in grams) of crude MAb produced per animal or acre?
i) Can the transgenic system perform the appropriate post-translational modifications?

4.3   Cost-related questions

a) What are the research and development costs related to development of the founder animal or plant?
b) What are the capital costs (primarily for land, barns, equipment) associated with each level of production from pilot scale through peak production?
c) What is the cost per gram to produce the recombinant MAb in pilot scale?
d) What is the cost per gram to produce the recombinant MAb at the various key production levels throughout the scale-up to peak production?
e) How will the downstream processing costs of a transgenic starting material compare to the costs from traditional feedstreams?

5. CONCLUSION

Traditional methods for biomanufacturing (*e.g.* mammalian cell culture and fermentation) will not be able to keep pace with the growing number of biopharmaceutical products being developed around the world. Transgenics shows great promise for large-scale biomanufacturing. Some believe that transgenics will not only alleviate the biomanufacturing capacity shortage, but will become the dominant biomanufacturing paradigm.

There are currently more than 10 transgenic species/systems that have either demonstrated the ability to produce MAbs, or show great promise of doing so. All of these systems can reasonably be expected to be scaled-up for the annual production of 100+ kilogram quantities of Mabs at costs that are competitive with, or favourable to those from traditional biomanufacturing methods.

New transgenic systems will almost certainly enter this arena, and some of the systems described in this chapter may ultimately prove to be unsuccessful. Nonetheless, the great diversity of the various transgenic systems described nearly guarantees that one or more of these systems will be approved by the relevant regulatory agencies for the production of therapeutic MAbs.

REFERENCES

Biotechnology Industry Organization website: www.bio.org

Li-Chan, E., Powrie, W., and Nakai, S., 1995, The Chemistry of Eggs and Egg Products. In *Egg Science and Technology, Fourth Edition* (Stadelman, W., and Cotterill, O., eds.), Haworth Press, New York, pp. 105-175.

Stadelman, W., 1995, Egg-Production Practices. In *Egg Science and Technology, Fourth Edition* (Stadelman, W., and Cotterill, O., eds.), Haworth Press, New York, pp. 9-37.

Sugino, H., Nitoda, T., and Juneja, L., 1997, General Chemical Composition of Hen Eggs. In *Hen Eggs: Their Basic and Applied Science* (Yamamoto, T., Juneja, L., Hatta, H., and Kim, M., eds.), CRC Press, Florida, pp. 13-24.

Chapter 2

GENERATION, ENGINEERING AND PRODUCTION OF HUMAN ANTIBODIES USING HuCAL®*

Ralf Ostendorp, Christian Frisch, and Margit Urban
MorphoSys AG, Lena-Christ-Strasse 48, D-82152 Martinsried/Planegg, Germany

1. INTRODUCTION

1.1 Antibody Libraries and Phage Display

It is almost three decades since Köhler and Milstein published their work on the use of cell fusion for the production of monoclonal antibodies from immunized mice (Köhler & Milstein, 1975). The technique was rapidly and widely adopted and has provided an enormous repertoire of useful research reagents (Little *et al.*, 2000). On the other hand, these antibodies have had limited success in human therapy (Glennie & Johnson, 2000). One reason is that murine antibodies often cause immune response in humans and lead to the generation of human anti-mouse antibodies (HAMA reaction), limiting the efficacy in long term and repeated administration (Jaffers *et al.*, 1986; Schellekens, 2002). Only in certain indications, *e.g.* for the treatment of immuno-suppressed cancer patients, murine antibodies can be used. Two examples are the radioisotope conjugated murine anti-CD20 antibodies Bexxar® (tositumomab) and Zevalin™ (ibritumomab), which are both applied for treatment of lymphoma. The development of genetic engineering has allowed the conversion of existing mouse monoclonal antibodies into chimeric mouse-human antibodies, and humanised molecules where only the

---

* Human Combinatorial Antibody Library

Antibodies, Volume 2: Novel Technologies and Therapeutic Use
Edited by G. Subramanian, Kluwer Academic/Plenum Publishers, New York 2004

complementarity-determining regions (CDR) are of murine origin (Queen *et al.*, 1989). To date, 13 therapeutic antibodies have obtained regulatory approval. Nowadays it is also possible to generate fully human antibodies, using either transgenic mice (Kellermann & Green, 2002), or *in vitro* technologies like phage display (Kretzschmar & von Rüden, 2002), ribosomal display (Hanes *et al.*, 2001), bacterial display (Chen & Georgiou, 2002) or yeast display (Boder & Wittrup, 2000). The generation of human antibodies by phage display methods has evolved as a powerful alternative for the generation of human antibodies for research, clinical and therapeutic applications. Phage display has become the most robust, and by far the most widely used *in vitro* technology for the selection of antibodies. Besides enabling the identification of antibodies in a fast, high-throughput mode, which allows comprehensive protein expression analyses, phage display has been used to identify fully human therapeutic antibodies. Recently, the first phage display-derived antibody, Humira™ (adalimumab; Lorenz, 2002) for the treatment of rheumatoid arthritis has received market approval by the US Food and Drug Administration (FDA). Moreover, about 30% of all fully human antibodies now in clinical development have been generated by this technology.

In phage display, the coupling of genotype and phenotype is usually accomplished by a genetic fusion of the gene of interest, *e.g.*, an antibody fragment, with one of the phage coat protein genes, usually gene III, of the *E. coli* bacteriophage fd or M13. Assembly of the phage and packaging of the phage or phagemid DNA takes place in *E. coli*. Hence, the genetic information coding for the fusion gene and the expressed fusion protein displayed on the surface of the phage are coupled.

Phage display libraries of human antibodies have usually been generated by PCR amplification of antibody genes from immunized donors (Barbas & Burton, 1996), germline sequences (Griffiths *et al.*, 1994, Jirholt *et al.*, 1998, Söderlind *et al.*, 2000) or naïve B-cell Ig repertoires (Vaughan *et al.*, 1996, Sheets *et al.*, 1998, de Haard *et al.*, 1999). Selection of these libraries by phage display has yielded human antibodies against numerous haptens, peptides and proteins. Immune libraries derived from IgG genes of immunized donors have the disadvantage that antibodies can only be made against the antigens used for immunization. In contrast, antibodies against virtually any antigen, including self, non-immunogenic or toxic antigens, can efficiently be isolated from non-immune libraries. The success of obtaining high-affinity antibodies is generally assumed to be related to the initial library size (Perelson, 1989). Therefore many attempts have been undertaken to make the library size as big as possible, and site-specific recombination systems have been created to overcome the library size limitations given by the conventional cloning strategies (Griffiths *et al.*, 1994, Sblattero *et al.*, 2000). However, in the libraries described above, the functional library size, *i.e.* the number of correctly assembled and functionally displayed clones, can be orders of magnitude below the apparent diversity usually reported, due to the applied technique of isolating and assembling the antibody genes from human material. Moreover, the restricted engineering possibilities in existing libraries made it desirable to use a complete protein engineering approach for the construction of human antibody libraries.

1.2 HuCAL® (Human Combinatorial Antibody Library)

The HuCAL® technology (see Figure 2.1) is a unique and innovative concept for the *in vitro* generation of highly specific and fully human antibodies. It focuses on a high number of correct antibody fragments, thus emphasizing on the functional and not on the apparent library size (Knappik *et al.*, 2000). In the HuCAL® libraries the structural diversity of the human antibody repertoire is represented by seven heavy chain and seven light chain variable region genes. The combination of these genes gives rise to 49 frameworks in the master library. The genes were optimised for expression and folding in *E. coli*. By superimposing highly variable genetic cassettes (CDRs) on these frameworks, the human antibody repertoire is perfectly reproduced. The genes and CDRs were prepared and assembled by chemical synthesis. A high functional quality of the library is guaranteed by diversifying the CDR regions with trinucleotide mixtures (Virnekäs *et al.*, 1994). The use of this trinucleotide mutagenesis (TRIM) technology allows the synthesis of any desired mixture of amino acids at will at every single position of the variable regions. Therefore, in HuCAL® libraries the length and the amino acid composition of the CDR regions are retained according to the natural antibody sequences found in humans. The analysis of a large database of rearranged human antibodies was the basis for the CDR design. The ratio of the amino acids found at each CDR position was reproduced in the respective trinucleotide mixture used for oligonucleotide synthesis. Amino acid residues not found at certain CDR positions in this database were not included in the trinucleotide mixtures at these positions. Hence, all HuCAL® CDRs reflect the natural composition of human CDRs. The modular design of the library with unique restriction sites flanking the CDR and framework regions, as well as compatible vector modules facilitate i) conversion into different antibody formats, ii) addition of effector functions and iii) further antibody optimisation by exchanging the CDR regions of selected binders by pre-built CDR libraries. The first HuCAL® library was constructed in the scFv format with both LCDR3 and HCDR3 diversified (Knappik *et al.*, 2000). Recently, a new version of the HuCAL® library, HuCAL®-Fab 1, was generated (Rauchenberger *et al.*, 2003), wherein we combined all the characteristics of the HuCAL® concept with the superior features of the Fab antibody format (see below).

HuCAL® GOLD is the latest and most powerful antibody library developed by MorphoSys (see Kretzschmar & von Rüden, 2002, and www.morphosys.com for more details). In addition to the proven advantages of the Fab format, we have included an entirely new selection technology, our proprietary CysDisplay™ (see below). In this library all six CDRs, *i.e.*, the complete antigen binding site, have been simultaneously diversified using the TRIM technology. The large diversity of the library (1.6×10^{10} members) facilitates the successful generation of high-quality antibodies.

CysDisplay™ is a novel and efficient display technology for selecting high affinity binders from antibody libraries using filamentous phage (Löhning, 2001). The method is based on the simultaneous periplasmic expression of engineered phage coat proteins and antibody fragments, both containing an unpaired cystein residue. Disulfide bond formation between both partners results in the formation of a protein complex and subsequent incorporation of this complex into phage particles, leading to the monovalent display of functional antibody fragments on the surface of phage (Figure 2.2). Since the disulfide linkage between the antibody fragment and the phage coat protein pIII is sensitive to reducing agents, an efficient elution protocol for the recovery of phages displaying specific, high affinity antibody fragments is available. This elution protocol can be applied to any type of antigen and is therefore ideally suited for high throughput applications.

Since all HuCAL® libraries proved well suited for selecting antibodies, and since the antibodies are very efficiently expressed in *E. coli*, procedures for the automated panning (AutoPan®) and screening (AutoScreen®) with high-throughput could be developed. The selection process of HuCAL® antibodies was simplified, miniaturised and parallelised using a modular system of specialised workstations which enables parallel and interlaced handling of work packages (AutoCAL™; Krebs *et al.*, 2001). This automated system allows the generation of high quality, validated and sequenced antibodies in a high-throughput fashion against hundreds of different antigens.

Whereas the large size and the high quality of our antibody libraries facilitate the selection of antibodies against virtually any given target in the initial panning process, it is the modularity of the master genes in combination with the customised expression vectors, which allows the selected antibody candidate(s) being engineered individually to the requested

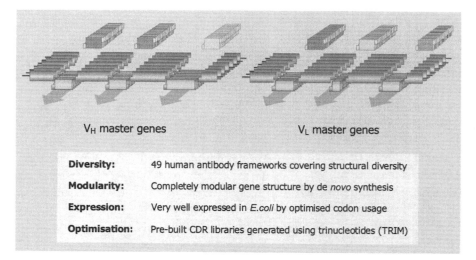

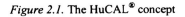

V_H master genes V_L master genes

Diversity:	49 human antibody frameworks covering structural diversity
Modularity:	Completely modular gene structure by de *novo* synthesis
Expression:	Very well expressed in *E.coli* by optimised codon usage
Optimisation:	Pre-built CDR libraries generated using trinucleotides (TRIM)

Figure 2.1. The HuCAL® concept

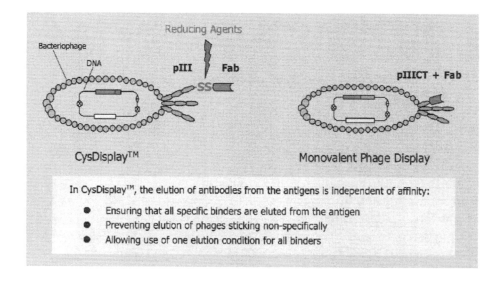

Reducing Agents

Bacteriophage

DNA   pIII   Fab   pIIICT + Fab

CysDisplay™   Monovalent Phage Display

In CysDisplay™, the elution of antibodies from the antigens is independent of affinity:

- Ensuring that all specific binders are eluted from the antigen
- Preventing elution of phages sticking non-specifically
- Allowing use of one elution condition for all binders

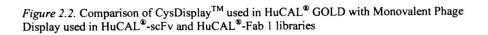

Figure 2.2. Comparison of CysDisplay™ used in HuCAL® GOLD with Monovalent Phage Display used in HuCAL®-scFv and HuCAL®-Fab 1 libraries

needs. Starting from the "lead" Fab fragment, selected from several billions of different members of the HuCAL® library, a rapid switch into a range of different antibody format(s) is easily accomplished (see section 2). There is a choice of different antibody formats, such as scFv, Fab or bivalent, tetravalent and multifunctional miniantibodies, as well as complete immunoglobulines, having in common the identical VH and VL genes (Figure 2.3). In addition, one can choose among a large variety of affinity tags or a combination thereof for protein purification or detection *in vitro* on the protein level (*e.g.* immunoassays, immunoblots, immunoprecipitation, capture based assays), on cells (*e.g.* FACS, immunocytochemistry), on tissues (*e.g.* immunohistochemistry) or even *in vivo* using customised conjugated chemicals or enzymes. The unique restriction sites of the HuCAL® system enable a rapid and customised optimisation of affinity and specificity of the lead candidate, starting from a single binder or a pool of initial binders and pre-made TRIM-diversified CDR-modules (see section 4.2).

2.   HuCAL® ANTIBODY FORMATS AND MANUFACTURING

2.1   The need for various antibody formats in clinical applications

During selection of an antibody candidate to be further developed as a drug substance, various parameters of the molecule are to be evaluated. Key topics to be addressed are i) the nature of the antibody (murine, chimeric, humanised, fully human), ii) the antibody format (immunoglobulin, fragment, conjugate), iii) target specificity, iv) the mode of interaction with the antigen, v) the affinity to the target antigen and vi) the anticipated biological function of the antibody (*e.g* blocking, signalling, targeting) (Waldmann *et al.*, 2000; Breedveld, 2000; Reichert, 2002; Gura, 2002).

Protein engineering has opened the door for a variety of alternative opportunities for treatment of diseases. The generation of bispecific antibodies for example has evolved from the laborious and sophisticated hybrid hybridoma ("quadroma") technology (Milstein & Cuello, 1983) to the straightforward and rapid microbial production of bispecific diabodies (Holliger *et al.*, 1993; Kiprianov *et al.*, 1999), miniantibodies (Plückthun & Pack, 1997) and combinations thereof (Lu *et al.*, 2002). Bispecific antibodies nowadays usually originate from a genetic or chemical fusion of two antibody fragments. A potent technology (BiTE™) was recently developed, capturing T-cells (*i.e.* surface antigens thereof) with one arm of a bispecific single chain antibody fragment and at the same time targeting cancer cells using the other one, thus promoting an efficient T-cell induced killing of cancer cells (Dreier *et al.*, 2002). If Fc-mediated functions are required, efficient technologies for the production of bispecific IgGs have also been developed (Carter, 2001).

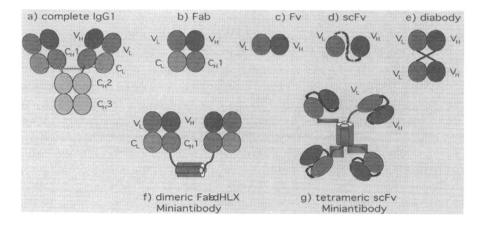

Figure 2.3. The modular structure of antibody derivatives. a) IgG1: complete immunoglobulin molecule; b) Fab: antigen-binding fragment; c) Fv: variable domain fragment; d) scFv: single chain variable domain fragment; e) Diabody: dimeric single chain variable domain fragment; f) Fab-dHLX Miniantibody: dimeric antigen-binding fragment; g) scFv-p53 Miniantibody: tetrameric single chain variable domain fragment.

Similarly, immunoconjugates are available, harbouring antigen specific binding sites for targeting and in addition covalently linked toxins, drugs, enzymes, dyes or radionuclides, dependent on the application in diagnostics or therapy. Those conjugates facilitate the efficient targeted delivery of effector functions to the antigen of interest. Although efficient, significant costs and major hurdles in the manufacturing and regulatory approval of these molecules must be considered, in order to obtain molecules of suitable size, stability, affinity and safety. Successful examples are the development of Zevalin™ (ibritumomab), the first approved radiolabeled antibody for cancer imaging and therapy (Grillo-Lopez, 2002), and Mylotarg™ (gemtuzumab), an antibody against the cellular surface antigen CD33, conjugated with the cytotoxic antibiotic calicheamicinan (Voutsadakis, 2002). Furthermore, for diagnostic purposes immunoconjugates can facilitate the non-invasive localization of tumours or other targets (Ramjiawan *et al.*, 2000).

Multivalent antibody fragments derive from genetic engineering of antibody fragments fused to multimerisation domains by recombinant DNA technology. These proteins can be produced efficiently in microorganisms

(Horn *et al.*, 1996). The obvious potential benefit in therapeutic applications is an improved *in vivo* targeting potential, caused by the increased functional affinity (avidity). In addition, the increased molecular weight is favourable in terms of serum clearance since larger molecules cannot easily pass the renal filtration threshold and remain longer in blood circulation. Miniantibodies have been proven very useful in research applications as well as in clinical applications (Holliger & Hoogenboom, 1998). As an example, the efficacy of miniantibodies was recently demonstrated in an *in vivo* study on tumour targeting (Willuda *et al.*, 2001). For monitoring of the antibodies *in vivo*, monomeric scFv, dimeric scFv-dHLX and tetrameric scFv-p53 miniantibodies could be efficiently radiolabelled with [99m]technetium-tricarbonyl. The labelled multimers all retained their state of oligomerisation, remained functional to at least 80% and showed better serum stability at 37°C than the monomer. The multimers dissociated significantly slower from the tumour antigen. Interestingly, in these assays a difference in avidity was not observed for the dimeric and tetrameric antibodies, since probably not more than two antigen molecules on the cell surface can be accessed simultaneously by one antibody molecule. However, the increasing degree of multimerisation did correlate with longer serum half-lives in blood. The tetrameric antibody revealed the best tumour targeting potential, 6-fold higher than its dimeric counterpart, and remained stably bound at the tumour, with a tumour-to-blood ratio of 13.5:1 after two days.

Fab fragments, which do not have an Fc-part, have also gained importance in clinical applications. Depending on the specific indication, it is often favourable to omit interactions with Fc-receptor bearing cells. The reduced molecular weight of the Fab favours efficient tissue penetration and fast body clearance. As described, the latter effect can be modified by choosing multivalent formats (Humphreys *et al.*, 1998, 2001; Willuda *et al.*, 2001; Weir *et al.*, 2002) and/or by chemical engineering, *e.g.* conjugation with polyethylene glycol (PEG) (Chapman *et al.*, 1999, 2002). In a recent study, an anti-TNFα Fab fragment was chemically engineered by site-specific PEGylation and subsequently evaluated in a pharmacokinetic study *in vivo* (Choy *et al.*, 2002). Compared to a TNFα-blocking IgG, the modified Fab fragment equally fulfilled the crucial requirements for *in vivo* administration, such as long plasma half-life, high affinity and safety. Whereas IgGs are produced in mammalian cell culture, Fab fragments can be produced in microorganisms and therefore represent a cost-attractive alternative to IgGs. Further examples for therapeutic antibody fragments having proven efficacy in clinical trials are the marketed chimeric Fab ReoPro™ (abciximab) and the two scFv fragments pexelizumab and H11, both in clinical development. The ReoPro™ Fab fragment was approved for human use in 1994 and has been administered to well over one million patients worldwide ever since. Considerable information has been accumulated about pharmacology, safety and efficacy (Davis *et al.*, 2000), a valuable starting point for further developments of therapeutic antibody fragments.

In summary, a significant need exists to evaluate optimised therapeutical approaches by comparing various antibody candidates in different formats mediating different strategies of treatments in early phases of drug development. Since the majority of candidates is not reaching clinical phases, it is mandatory to limit costs by shortening timelines for an efficient candidate screening early on. Ideally, a panel of antibody candidates will be evaluated, targeting different epitopes of the same antigen or targeting the same epitope with different intrinsic or functional affinities or triggering different Fc-mediated effector functions *in vivo* (Mimura *et al.*, 2001; Jefferis *et al.*, 1998, Jefferis & Lund, 2002). Such requirements are accomplished most efficiently by using a *"plug & play"* system, which keeps the antigen specific regions of the "parent" antibody untouched throughout conversion into different antibody formats. The combination of modularity and fully human design makes HuCAL® a unique source for such antibody-based applications ranging from high-throuput screening all the way to therapeutic antibodies.

In the following, the various HuCAL® antibody formats will be introduced, and examples for the application of the HuCAL® technology in target research and for the generation of therapeutic antibodies will be given.

2.2 Monovalent and multivalent HuCAL® antibody fragments

Unlike the traditional immunoglobulin format of 2 heavy chains (4 domains each, VH-CH1-CH2-CH3) and 2 light chains (2 domains each, VL-CL), the Fab fragment only consists of 2 chains, the heavy chain fragment Fd (VH-CH1) and the light chain (VL-CL), lacking the Fc-part (CH2-CH3), which is usually post-translationally modified with complex sugar residues (Figure 2.3). In the HuCAL®-Fab format, no intermolecular disulfide bonds are present, since the respective cystein residues were omitted. The Fab fragments can easily be produced as monomeric soluble molecules, which is a crucial pre-requisite for enabling a reliable screening of intrinsic affinities. In the HuCAL®-scFv format, VH and VL are covalently linked by a peptide linker of 20 amino acid residues. As for multivalent antibody fragments, the term "miniantibody" was used as a synonym for miniaturised antibodies engineered to mimic complete immunoglobulins in terms of multivalent binding with similar spacing and rotational freedom of the variable domain arms, but at the same time lacking the Fc-part, thus reducing the molecular weight of the molecule significantly (Pack & Plückthun, 1992; Plückthun & Pack, 1997). HuCAL® miniantibodies have been successfully produced as non-covalently linked dimeric and tetrameric molecules, which spontaneously assemble in a soluble and functional form in the periplasm of *E. coli* (Pack *et al.*, 1993; Krebs *et al.*, 2001). Dimerisation and tetramerisation was easily facilitated by genetically connecting the antibody fragment modules with the synthetic helix-turn-helix domain "dHLX" (O'Shea *et al.*, 1989) or with the multimerisation domain of the human p53 protein (Rheinnecker *et al.*, 1996), respectively. The synthetic dHLX dimerisation domain is very small (3 kDa) and dimerises in an anti-parallel orientation to a four-helix-bundle giving the two non-covalently dimerising Fab fragments the Y-like shape of a bivalent antibody. For scFv-dHLX constructs, functional affinities were obtained, identical to the complete parent immunoglobulin (Pack *et al.*, 1993, 1995). Although in general a reduction in production yield can be observed, as compared with monovalent fragments, it has been shown that functional miniantibodies can efficiently be produced from optimised high cell density *E. coli* cultures in the gram per litre range (Pack *et al.*, 1993; Horn *et al.*, 1996).

2.3   Biophysical properties of HuCAL® antibody fragments

The importance of the biophysical properties of clinically relevant antibody candidates has recently been demonstrated for a high affinity scFv fragment raised against the tumour-associated antigen EGP-2 (epithelial glycoprotein-2) (Willuda *et al.*, 1999). Despite its high antigen binding capacity *in vitro*, the scFv failed to efficiently enrich on tumours *in vivo*. Due to an insufficient thermodynamic stability, the antibody had to be engineered by CDR grafting and point mutation approaches, before the desired functionality *in vivo* was obtained.

In order to evaluate the biophysical properties of HuCAL® antibodies in more detail, a comprehensive study was recently performed on the isolated seven HuCAL® consensus VH and VL domains and compared to combinations thereof in the scFv format (Ewert *et al.*, 2003a). The key parameters, that influence solubility, folding efficiency and stability of the isolated domains and the scFv constructs were identified. Since each antibody domain represents a consensus sequence of a human variable antibody domain, the properties of the HuCAL® constructs may be extrapolated to all human antibodies. The studies confirm earlier observations, that many de-/stabilising effects contribute to the overall intrinsic stability of a protein by a complex pattern of intra- and intermolecular electrostatic and hydrophobic interactions among amino acid side chains, secondary structure elements and domain interfaces (Brandts *et al.*, 1988; Matthews, 1995; Jaenicke *et al.*, 1996; Jaenicke & Lilie, 2000). As for the scFv fragments, certain CDRs turned out to have a strong influence on the packing of the hydrophobic core and thus on the overall stability of the domains. Likewise, the core residues exert a strong influence on the conformation of the CDRs, which in turn determine affinity and specificity of the antibody. Not surprisingly, the combination of the most stable VH domain with the most stable VL domain resulted in a very stable scFv fragment VH3Vκ3. However, the most stable scFvs originate from Vλ domains, which represent the least stable domains, when isolated. This cooperative effect is probably due to the stabilising impact of the domain interfaces in concert with the CDRs contributing to an improved packing of the hydrophobic core. These physicochemical studies together with further rational protein engineering approaches have meanwhile identified and further improved the "weakest links" within antibody structures, providing the proof-of-concept, that any antibody construct can be engineered to the desired application (Forsberg *et al.*, 1997; Wall & Plückthun, 1999; Wörn & Plückthun, 1999, 2001; Ewert *et al.*, 2003b). The essentials of these and other studies have been implemented in the HuCAL® GOLD antibody library.

In order to evaluate the stabilities of different Fab constructs with identical target specificity, a comparison between a mouse Fab, a chimeric Fab (mouse CL-CH1 + human VL-VH) and a fully human HuCAL® Fab was performed. In addition, three constructs were designed where intermolecular disulfide bonds between the respective heavy and light chains were introduced (unpublished results; B. Brocks, R. Ostendorp). The six constructs were produced in *E. coli* and subsequently incubated at 37°C in human plasma for up to 15 days and at up to 70°C in buffer for 30 min. In terms of expression yields, an additional intermolecular disulfide bond between heavy and light chain only had a beneficial impact on the mouse construct, whereas the chimeric and human Fab fragments showed a clearly worse expression, thus confirming earlier observations on the reduced expression and folding efficiency of disulfide linked antibody fragments in *E. coli* (Humphreys *et al.*, 1997; Schmiedl *et al.*, 2000). Stability testing of the purified proteins at 37°C in human plasma showed no significant decrease in binding activity over an incubation time of up to 15 days.

Elevated temperature studies also serve as indicators for the intrinsic stability of proteins. As shown in Figure 2.4, the mouse constructs clearly represent the least stable formats. As for the disulfide bonds, it is only at very high temperatures, where a stabilising impact on the chimeric and human constructs can be observed, an additional ~20% activity can be retained using disulfide-stabilised constructs. These data indicate, that

HuCAL® Fab fragments are likely to be equally suited for *in vivo* applications as disulfide bonded constructs are. Due to the absence of an intermolecular disulfide bond in HuCAL® Fab fragments, there is neither the risk of wrong disulfides or multimers to be formed during protein folding and assembly nor can disulfide shuffling occur in the "mature" protein. However, in case an intermolecular disulfide bond is needed, it can easily be engineered into the HuCAL® construct.

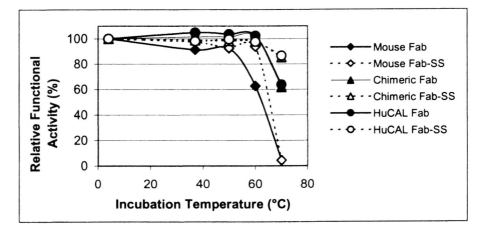

Figure 2.4. The impact of antibody format (mouse, chimeric, human) and an intermolecular disulfide bond (SS) on the heat stability of Fab constructs

In a different study, the applicability of HuCAL® antibodies for analytical and diagnostic applications was evaluated. HuCAL®-Fab fragments were generated against a panel of bacterial toxins as markers for pathogenic microorganisms (unpublished results; K. Kramer, Technical University of Munich, Germany). In addition, haptens like insecticides and herbicides were used as antigens. As compared to "conventional" immunization approaches yielding IgG-derived polyclonal antibodies, highly specific HuCAL®-Fab fragments could be generated with superior features in terms of specificity and robustness. For example, the sensitivity of the Fab fragments in herbicide detection showed an up to 30.000-fold better performance compared to their polyclonal counterparts. Since robustness against unfavourable extrinsic factors like organic solvents and elevated temperatures is a pre-requisite for the employment of "biosensors" in analytical applications, the Fab fragments were also tested under these conditions. For most of the candidates, an incubation in 53% (v/v) methanol did not affect their analytical potential significantly. Similarly, selected HuCAL® antibodies have even retained full binding activity upon incubation at up to 80°C for 24 hours.

These findings confirm, that the design of the HuCAL®-Fab constructs has been optimised regarding protein folding, framework stability and expression yields. Heavy and light chains can efficiently fold and assemble in the periplasmic space of *E. coli*, without necessitating a stabilising intermolecular disulfide bond. Nevertheless, the resulting β-sandwich structure still leaves sufficient flexibility in the Fab molecule to efficiently bind the antigen of interest. Thus, an optimised combination of high intrinsic stability, stable non-covalent association of heavy and light chains and reliable functionality has been realised in the HuCAL®-Fab construct.

2.4   Immunoglobulins

In the recent years several therapeutic antibodies, mostly IgG molecules, have been approved for clinical applications (Glennie & Johnson, 2000; Reichert, 2001, 2002). The "renaissance" of antibodies as therapeutics is accelerated by the phage display technology, which allows a much faster generation of specific human antibodies than the conventional techniques. The selection and characterisation of human Fab fragments from the large antibody repertoire of the HuCAL® GOLD library can be performed within weeks, even for toxic, low immunogenic or self antigens and the modularity of the HuCAL® system allows the rapid conversion of the selected Fab into immunoglobulins. HuCAL® vectors for the expression of fully human IgG1, IgG4 and IgA1 are currently available. IgG1 as the predominant immunoglobulin in human serum promotes phagocytosis, antibody-dependent cellular cytotoxicity and superoxide generation of diverse cell populations by preferential binding to all three types of Fcγ–receptors (Gessner *et al.*, 1998). In combination with its complement binding activity, IgG1 is most often leading to a depletion of target cells (Mourad *et al.*, 1998). In contrast, the IgG4 subclass is rather weakly binding to Fcγ–receptors and shows a low complement fixing capacity (Bachelez *et al.*, 1998). Therefore, targeted cells are not depleted but mainly coated. The predominantly bivalent serum IgA1 does not bind to C1q (Morton *et al.*, 1993), but is capable of activating the alternative complement pathway. It binds to Fcα receptors thereby promoting phagocytosis, superoxide generation and clearance of immune complexes (Carayannopoulos *et al.*, 1994).

HuCAL® vectors for the expression of chimeric human/mouse IgG1, IgG2a and IgG3 are also available. The chimeric antibodies, harbouring murine Fc-parts, serve as useful tools in preclinical animal studies and in immunohistochemistry on human tissues, as the endogenous human immunoglobulins often cause background staining. The chimeric constructs with their murine constant regions can easily be detected in a human protein background.

The conversion of any HuCAL® Fab into the format with the desired effector function is performed by two simple cloning steps, omitting any PCR steps in between that might cause mutations in the fully human sequences. The constant region genes in the Ig-vectors harbour silent mutations to remove restriction enzyme sites non-compatible with the modular design of HuCAL®. Thus HuCAL® allows seamless "switching" of Ig-classes or –subclasses at any stage of the development.

2.5   Antibody manufacturing

As for the production of antibody fragments, protein engineering has opened the way to circumvent the laborious and time-consuming generation of Fab fragments by proteolytic digestion of full IgG molecules produced in cell culture. Since the first antibody fragments have been functionally expressed in *E. coli* (Skerra & Plückthun, 1988; Better *et al.*, 1988), they are nowadays preferably produced in microorganisms. In general, microbial systems, such as bacteria, yeast and fungi represent the most mature production processes for biopharmaceuticals. Even for laboratory-scale production of research material, impressive yields in the range of multi-grams of soluble and functional antibody fragment per litre of high cell density growth cultures have been reported (Horn *et al.*, 1996; Plückthun *et al.*, 1996; Humphreys *et al*, 2002).

The main advantages of microbial manufacturing are i) the applicability to any production scale from micrograms to kilograms of material, ii) known bioprocessing procedures, iii) very high product yields, iv) favourable timelines and v) attractive costs of goods. Recent estimates have calculated a cost factor of 3 to 10 in favour of large-scale bacterial production systems as compared with mammalian ones (UBS Warburg). For these reasons and despite the fact that the majority of marketed therapeutic antibodies are mammalian cell culture derived IgGs, major efforts and investments are currently being made in order to increase production capacity for microbial fermentation. A major task is the establishment of generic fermentation and downstream processes for antibody fragments, comparable to the well-established IgG-pipelines. The importance of this task is underlined by the fact, that downstream processing accounts for about 50% of the overall manufacturing costs in microbial processes. A first step in this direction has been made by the establishment of a heat precipitation step during downstream processing of *E. coli* derived Fab fragments (Weir & Bailey, 1997), making use of the high intrinsic stability of this antibody format (see also section 2.3).

For expression and folding in *E. coli*, the codon usage of the HuCAL® VH and VL master genes as well as of the constant region genes CH1, Cλ and Cκ were optimised (Knappik *et al.*, 2000). Therefore, high yields of HuCAL® antibody fragments can routinely be achieved from standardised *E. coli* expression cultures. Although the codon usage was brought in line with bacterial expression, disadvantages for the expression of HuCAL® antibodies in mammalian cells have not been observed, indicating that the codons are not compromising mammalian expression. The HuCAL® Ig-vector design is in principle suited for i) transient expression, ii) stable expression with episomal maintenance of the heterologous DNA and iii) stable expression with chromosomal maintenance of the heterologous DNA. The Ig-vectors enable to generate sufficient material for the evaluation of the immunoglobulins very rapidly, as the yields from non-optimised standardised small-scale expression and affinity purification range from 5 to 15 mg per litre static culture supernatant (Krebs *et al.*, 2001). By applying more sophisticated cell culture methods in combination with high yielding host/vector systems the yields in IgG production are drastically improved. Yields of more than 0.5 g functional IgG per litre culture supernatant have been obtained. The defined HuCAL® antibody frameworks, which exhibit uniform expression and folding behaviour, should allow generic manufacturing pipelines to be established.

2.6   Emerging technologies for antibody manufacturing

Despite the fact that efficient manufacturing procedures for antibodies have been developed, both in microbial and mammalian host cell systems, several drawbacks can be observed, such as incorrect protein folding or glycosylation, inclusion body formation, proteolytic degradation or toxicity of the recombinant protein for the host cell. However, inclusion body formation has been exploited as an elegant "concentration step" of the recombinant target protein already within the host cell. This simplifies subsequent downstream processes significantly, but on the other hand also requires sophisticated refolding steps to be established (Buchner & Rudolph, 1991). As for the other potential drawbacks, a trend towards the combination of protein engineering of the antibody with "metabolic engineering" of the host cell can currently be observed. Optimisation of the translational level of the recombinant protein (Simmons & Yansura, 1996) or knock-out of entire host cell genes, coding for cell death enhancing proteins (Tey *et al.*, 2000) have been shown to increase product yield and lifetime of the host cells, respectively. Manipulation of the intracellular redox system by co-secretion of chaperones and disulfide isomerases or the addition of low molecular weight supplements during fermentation have also increased the yields of soluble and functional protein significantly (Lilie *et al.*, 1993; Bothmann & Plückthun, 1998; Martineau *et al.*, 1998; Schäffner *et al.*, 2001; Venturi *et al.*, 2002; Laden *et al.*, 2002; Hiniker & Bardwell, 2003). In terms of limitations of species specific glycosylation patterns, this problem can also be abolished by metabolic engineering (Baker *et al.*, 2001; Bakker *et al.*, 2001), or alternative eukaryotic host cell lines (Palomares *et al.*, 2003).

In parallel to the "engineering approach", alternative prokaryotic and eukaryotic expression systems are currently being evaluated. For example, cell wall-less bacteria (L-forms), lacking the outer cell membrane, were employed for the production of scFv fragments and scFv-dHLX miniantibodies, which could be synthesised and correctly processed in the absence of a periplasmic compartment (Gumpert & Hoischen, 1998; Kujau *et al.*, 1998). L-form cells of *Proteus mirabilis* were used to express scFv fragments, which were of potential clinical interest, but showed severe production problems in *E. coli*. It turned out, that none of these problems occurred in *Proteus* and yields of up to 200 mg scFv per litre of culture medium were obtained (Rippmann *et al.*, 1998). Alternative human cell lines such as PER.C6 (Jones *et al.*, 2003) and HKB11 (Cho *et al.*, 2003) have recently gained interest, having the potential of providing superior expression yields and more favourable posttranslational modifications, which might positively affect immunogenicity of the antibodies. Since these human cell lines have been shown to function equally well at various production scales, they might also be able to overcome yet another bottleneck in drug development, namely the transition from screening scale material to large scale manufacturing.

Transgenic animals and plants represent an alternative, which might help overcoming an anticipated manufacturing capacity shortage. Although rather long lead times have to be accepted, major regulatory hurdles still have to be taken and the first "transgenic antibody" remains to be approved, it might become an attractive technology with respect to the cost of goods.

By expressing full-length IgG molecules in the *E. coli* periplasm (Simmons *et al.*, 2002), an elegant link has recently been established between microbial fermentation being the most mature technology for biopharmaceutical proteins in general and IgGs being the most successful biopharmaceutical antibody format. Antigen binding and pharmocokinetic properties remained unchanged in the aglycosylated IgG as compared with mammalian derived counterparts. This technology might become an attractive alternative for antibody applications, where glycosylation is dispensable.

With the ambitious goal to leave behind all the cell related problems in protein production, cell-free translation systems have been developed, mimicking the protein expression machinery *in vitro* (Spirin *et al.*, 1988).

With respect to antibody production *in vitro*, the effect of mRNA structure, amino acid sequence changes and protein labelling as well as the impact of extrinsic factors such as chaperones, disulfide isomerases or medium components on folding, assembly and functionality of antibody fragments have been examined for scFv fragments (Ryabova *et al.*, 1997; Kigawa *et al.*, 1999) and Fab fragments (Jiang *et al.*, 2002). Although cell free translation systems have recently evolved dramatically resulting in commercially available "kits", which already yield milligram amounts of protein, the potential and the economy of this technology for large scale manufacturing of antibodies *in vitro* remains to be shown (for a review see Jermutus *et al.*, 1998).

Whereas the "traditional" antibody manufacturing practices demonstrate proven success and thus represent a "paved way" for drug approval, the anticipated capacity needs of well over one million litre fermenter space in the next few years can probably not be met using conventional technologies (UBS Warburg). A recent study of the Center for Biologics Evaluation and Research (CBER) revealed, that delays in regulatory approvals of Biologics Licence Applications (BLA) most frequently can be related to manufacturing issues, followed by safety and efficacy issues (*BioCentury*, Feb. 3, 2003). This underlines the need for more efficient and/or alternative manufacturing strategies for compound supply. The accumulated knowledge about approved therapeutic proteins, combined with the recent advances in analytical methods will provide more detailed information about how to improve the manufacturing process. By rational design of the antibody, the expression system and the manufacturing processes, regulatory approvals will be more streamlined in the future. However, any new system for improved antibody expression has to face the (regulatory) risk of "being the first of its kind" in clinical trials.

3. HuCAL® – APPLICATIONS IN TARGET RESEARCH

3.1 Antibodies against EST-encoded polypeptides

Genome projects have identified a huge number of genes, accelerating the need for reagents to study the expression of these genes and to elucidate the function and cellular location of the gene products. *Expressed Sequence Tags* (ESTs) are gene fragments, which usually represent the first evidence for the existence and expression of a gene (Adams *et al.*, 1995). Although ESTs are generated in vast numbers as part of the Human Genome Project, the functions of the corresponding genes and gene products are mostly still unknown. Antibodies are the first choice tools to determine the level of expression of the EST-encoded protein in various tissues of the organism, and to finally elucidate its function. It was suggested earlier to express the ESTs and to generate antibodies by immunizing animals with the corresponding polypeptides (Venter & Adams, 1993). In a similar approach, DNA constructs comprising open reading frames have been injected into animals to generate an immune response against the polypeptide expressed *in vivo* (Sykes & Johnston, 1999). However, these approaches are not amenable to the high-throughput generation of antibodies.

We have developed a generally applicable method, designated HuCAL®-EST, for the high-throughput generation of antibodies to EST-encoded polypeptides. We express these polypeptides as fusions with the N1-domain of the gIII-protein of filamentous phage M13 in *E. coli* leading to high-level expression and formation of inclusion bodies. After standardised purification and refolding, these fusion proteins enter our high-throughput antibody generation process. The selected antibodies can then be employed for immunohistochemistry (IHC) experiments for target research/validation purposes (see section 3.2). The main advantages of this process are i) high-throughput, ii) fast delivery of antibodies raised against (unknown) protein fragments and recognising the maternal protein, iii) high numbers of IHC-grade antibodies recognising various epitopes of the maternal protein and iv) very good overall success rates. Alternatively, antibodies can be generated against peptides derived from an EST or protein sequence (Persic *et al.*, 1999; Krebs *et al.*, 2001). However, due to the relatively small contact region of the antigen binding site on the antibody with the small peptide, which limits the maximum binding energy, it is difficult to obtain anti-peptide antibodies with sufficiently high affinities. Moreover, to increase the probability of selection of binders recognising the maternal protein, antibodies against different peptides derived from one target sequence have to be generated (Siegel *et al.*, 2000). This causes a "target inflation", which represents a significant cost factor in target research. The use of long EST-encoded polypeptides, covalently linked to a well folding fusion partner as in HuCAL®-EST, in addition facilitates three-dimensional structures (*i.e.* epitopes) to be generated. As compared to short linear peptide antigens, the success rate to generate an antibody recognising the maternal protein of interest is significantly increased by the use of the HuCAL®-EST technology.

We have demonstrated the success of this method in a proof-of-principle study for eleven different N1-fusion proteins containing fragments of human Mac-1 alpha chain, MHC class II alpha and beta chain, NF-*k*B p50, ICAM-1 and the human cytomegalovirus protein UL84 (Frisch *et al.*, 2003).

Fragments of these well-characterised proteins have been chosen to evaluate the specificity of the generated antibodies on the respective maternal full-length proteins. Fusion proteins with molecular weights ranging from 19 kDa to 76 kDa could be rapidly expressed, purified and refolded to soluble proteins, even in the presence of transmembrane domains. The redox system routinely used for refolding of the fusion proteins enables disulfide bonds to be established. However, we have not tested the biological activity of the fusion proteins. The refolded protein preparation will probably consist of a mixture of correctly folded functional domains and misfolded inactive molecules. From a single panning process, we have selected antibodies that react either with the denatured, or the native maternal protein or with both of them. The suitability of "HuCAL® anti-EST antibodies" for target identification and target validation was proven in various methods, such as Western blotting, flow cytometry and IHC. The antibodies displayed affinities in the low nanomolar range. The HuCAL®-EST technology is now routinely used in a high throughput-mode for the generation of IHC-positive antibodies (see also Figure 2.5). To date, the success rates for selecting target-specific antibodies (including EST-encoded polypeptides, peptides and proteins), which work in Western Blot and immunohistochemistry is about 85% and 74%, respectively. Due to their fully human nature and modular design, these antibodies, initially evaluated in target identification and validation programs, may then immediately serve as lead candidates for drug development.

3.2   Protein expression profiling

In vitro methods such as Western blotting, FACS, immunopreciptitation, ELISA or array-based methods are routinely used for protein expression analysis. In addition, staining of tissues with specific antibodies has become a powerful method in the field of target identification and validation for *in situ* protein expression profiling. Traditionally (bivalent) IgGs have been the constructs of choice for IHC. We have established the bivalent Fab construct Fab-dHLX (see section 2.2), which proved to be ideally suited for applications in IHC (see Figures 2.3 and 2.5). Dimeric Fab-dHLX antibodies, mimicking full IgGs in terms of bivalency, can rapidly be produced in milligram amounts in *E. coli*, thus omitting time-consuming IgG production and therefore facilitating high-throughput IHC applications. With respect to seamless transitions of high-throughput pipelines, the Fab-dHLX format completes the entire way from antigen generation (HuCAL®-EST), antibody generation and production (AutoCAL™) to antibody selectivity screening. Novel targets, *e.g.* derived from genomics approaches, can now be validated by immunohistochemical studies at high speed within weeks

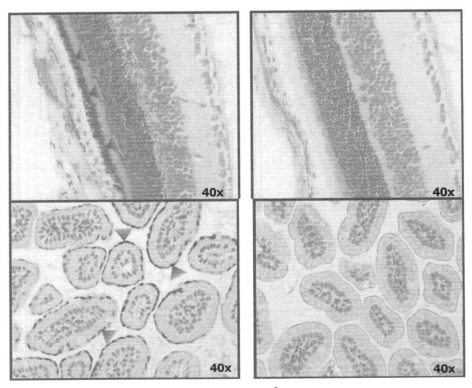

Figure 2.5. Immunohistochemistry using HuCAL® Fab-dHLX antibodies on paraffin-embedded tissue sections. Upper panel: cross-section mouse eye (retina); specific staining of the rod area (arrows). Lower panel: cross-section mouse small intestine (through intestine villi); specific staining of the columnar epithelial cells (arrows). EST-encoded polypeptides (256 and 150 amino acid residues, respectively) were produced using HuCAL®-EST technology. Specific antibodies were generated using the automated AutoCAL™ technology and subsequently produced in *E. coli*. Right panels represent negative controls.

and with very high quality (Sun C. *et al.*, 2003). Examples for successful applications of the proprietary bivalent Fab-dHLX format in IHC are shown in Figure 2.5. From bioinformatics approaches, open reading frames (ORFs) were identified in cDNA sequences, which potentially code for therapeutically relevant proteins. Milligram amounts of EST-encoded protein fragments were produced in   *E.coli* and subsequently used as antigens in our automated antibody generation process (AutoCAL™). Screening of the output then revealed antibodies, which facilitate validation of the target in IHC. Therefore, the assumed expression patterns of gene products based on cDNA studies can be confirmed experimentally on the protein level within a few weeks using HuCAL® -technologies.

3.3 Antibody microarrays

In target research and clinical diagnostics applications, antibody microarrays have become a useful tool for the simultaneous detection and quantification of various defined "marker" proteins within the proteome of the target cell. Innovative approaches for array-based high-throughput assays are currently being developed, ranging from the immobilisation of entire scFv-expressing bacteria (deWildt et al., 2000) or eukaryotic cells (Schwenk et al., 2002) to proteins/antibodies or fragments thereof (Luecking et al., 1999; Cahill, 2001; Haab et al., 2001; Eickhoff et al., 2002). The proven efficacy of antibodies in targeting and capturing of antigens has recently boosted their employment as receptors or biosensors on "bio-chips" (Lesley, 2001; Hayhurst, 2001; Joos et al., 2002; MacBeath, 2002; Templin et al., 2002; Walter et al., 2002). New immobilisation methods now facilitate the directed orientation of antibodies, increasing the fraction of functional molecules on the surface and thus the binding capacity of the "biosensor" (Peluso et al., 2003). Because of its reliable functionality and stability (see section 2.3) and the faster and cheaper production as compared to IgG, the Fab format again proves to be the format of choice for array-based applications.

We have further analysed the application of antibody microarrays for the reliable measurement of affinities. As described above, recombinant antibody technologies allow the isolation of binders to nearly any given target molecule within a few weeks, which indicates that the bottleneck in the generation of efficient lead molecules has therefore shifted from the selection and production process to the detailed characterisation of the antibodies. While established methods for affinity determination, such as surface plasmon resonance, which rely on kinetic measurements of association and dissociation constants, give reliable results with a reasonable consumption of sample, the speed of the methods is the limiting factor for screening purposes. Therefore, microarray approaches for the determination of relative affinities have an enormous potential to speed up the process of the characterisation of protein-protein interactions. Based on the predictable expression behaviour of HuCAL®-Fab fragments, we have therefore recently developed array-based technologies for reliable high-throughput parallel screening of Fab candidates. Starting from crude E. coli lysates, an efficient method for affinity screening was established (Joos et al., 2002; O. Poetz et al., in preparation). The goals were i) to quantify the amount of Fab fragments present in the crude lysates, ii) to simultaneously detect antigen specific binding of the Fab fragments as compared to irrelevant antigens (crossreactivity screening) and iii) to determine the apparent affinities of the antibody-antigen interactions. As confirmed by surface plasmon resonance measurements, the method is useful for a fast and reliable affinity ranking of minute amounts of non-purified Fab from small-scale *E. coli* cultures on minute amounts of antigen. Thus, the HuCAL® high-throughput antibody generation platform could be combined with a microarray-based high-throughput affinity ranking method. Applications of this method comprise an efficient library screening, *e.g.*, in target research programs, as well as proteomics and clinical diagnostics. Further developments in this direction are on the way.

3.4   Functional analyses

Beyond pure binding to the antigen, antibodies can exhibit functional activity via a variety of different mechanisms (for review see Glennie & Johnson, 2000). First of all the antibody can simply block specific activities or interactions, *e.g.* inhibition of enzyme activity, neutralisation of soluble mediators, or blocking interactions between ligand and receptor, cell and cell adhesion molecules, or virus and host cell. A whole range of different assays are established at MorphoSys to evaluate blocking potential of selected antibodies. An example for a protease inhibition assay is described in section 4.1.2, examples of protein-cell and cell-cell adhesion assays can be found in sections 4.1.3 and 4.1.4. In addition, antibodies can exhibit signalling function. Binding to cell surface receptors can trigger transmembrane signals that control the cell cycle and induce *e.g.* cell proliferation or cell death. In most cases, this requires cross-linking of the target molecules and therefore bivalent antibody formats are used. The antibodies substitute for specific ligands, which activate their receptor molecules by inducing receptor dimerisation and subsequent signalling pathways. Proliferation and killing assays are established and an example will be given in section 4.2.2. Full Ig molecules can also exhibit functional activity via induction of the immunological effector systems (see section 2.4). Induction of the classical pathway of complement activation results in complement-dependent cytotoxicity (CDC). Activation of effector cells via binding to the respective Fcγ receptors leads to antibody-dependent cell-mediated cytotoxicity (ADCC). Both mechanisms are induced by the human IgG1 subclass, while IgG4 is rather weakly binding to Fcγ–receptors and shows a low complement fixing capacity. HuCAL®-IgG1 has proven to be effective in both assay systems. Overall, antibodies originally generated by target research programs can directly be characterized for functional activity allowing a seamless transition to the identification of therapeutic antibodies.

4. HuCAL® – DESIGNED FOR THERAPEUTIC APPLICATION

4.1 Antibody generation

The HuCAL® technology is currently being exploited for the generation of therapeutic antibodies in a broad spectrum of indications, such as inflammation, leukemia, solid cancer as well as cardiovascular, liver, and CNS-related diseases. Therapeutically relevant HuCAL® antibodies were generated against a wide range of different target molecules, including adhesion proteins, receptor tyrosine kinases, MHC molecules, cytokines, proteases, and protease inhibitors. In this section examples will be given for antibody generation against the serine protease MT-SP1, the human fibroblast growth factor receptor 3 (FGFR3) and the human intercellular adhesion molecule 1 (ICAM-1). These examples demonstrate the broad applicability of the HuCAL® libraries with different antibody formats and selection strategies.

4.1.1 Selection procedure

The design of an appropriate selection strategy is crucial for the rapid generation of antibodies with therapeutic potential. Direct immobilisation of purified antigen to *e.g.* microtitre plates is used as simple and effective standard procedure, but can lead to conformational changes of the antigen. As a consequence not all isolated antibodies will bind to the native protein. For soluble factors, *e.g.* cytokines, the more favourable alternative is panning on antigen in solution (*e.g.* Hawkins *et al.*, 1992; Schier *et al.*, 1996a, b). For example, the antigen is biotinylated and bound phages are selected via capture to streptavidin-coated plates or beads. An important prerequisite is to prove that biotinylation of the antigen has no impact on its functionality. For cell surface expressed targets, panning on whole cells is the method of choice (*e.g.* Watters *et al.*, 1997; Hoogenboom *et al.*, 1999; Huls *et al.*, 1999). Cell surface proteins are often difficult or even impossible to purify, the antigen conformation can change significantly during purification and immobilisation, or the target proteins have not been characterized at all. Panning on cells guarantees that selection is focused on biologically relevant epitopes, taking homophilic or heterophilic interactions of the antigen on the cell surface into account. Both, differential cell panning with alternating rounds on purified antigen and cell-based antigen as well as pure cell pannings have been applied successfully with HuCAL® libraries (Marget *et al.*, 2000; Krebs *et al.*, 2001). Cell panning was for example employed for the human major histocompatibility class I (HLA class I) allele Cw*0602 as an antigen (Marget *et al.*, 2000). Eight different HuCAL®-scFv were isolated that recognise native antigen and can be readily used in flow cytometry and immunoprecipitation. All scFv fragments are highly specific for the defined HLA-I allele, and do not exhibit significant cross-reactivity with a panel of different class I alleles. The selected anti-HLA class I antibodies can be applied in tissue typing as well as for studies of disease association with HLA variants, as for example HLA-C in regulating natural killer cell activity in the context of recurrent miscarriages (King *et al.*, 1996a, b).

4.1.2   Application example: HuCAL® antibodies against serine protease MT-SP1

The membrane-type serine protease 1 (MT-SP1) is highly expressed in many human cancer-derived cell lines and has been implicated in extracellular matrix re-modelling, tumour growth, and metastasis (Lin *et al.*, 1999a, b; Takeuchi *et al.*, 2000; Hooper *et al.*, 2001). Specific reagents targeting MT-SP1 could be of great value for diagnosis, prognosis, and therapy of cancer. One obstacle in generation of specific inhibitors is the omnipresence of proteases in nature comprising approximately 2% of the entire human genome (Harris *et al.*, 2000). Similar active site elements hamper the generation of inhibitors selective for a particular protease.

To this end, Sun J. *et al.* (2003) screened the HuCAL®-scFv library against recombinant MT-SP1. To increase stringency of the panning process, the serine proteases inhibitor ecotin was added as competitor during washing procedure. Five antibody fragments could be selected with K_D values in the range of 160 pM to 1.8 nM as determined by surface plasmon resonance. *In vitro* potency was determined in inhibition assays with the human MT-SP1 protease domain resulting in apparent K_i values from 50 pM to 129 nM. Two of the antibodies revealed approximately 800- to 1500-fold selectivity when tested against mouse MT-SP1, which represents the most homologous serine protease family member with 86.6% sequence identity. For two scFv fragments no inhibition of the murine enzyme could be detected. One of the antibodies recognised MT-SP1 on human prostate tissue as well as on prostate cancer tissue in immunohistochemical studies. Interestingly, MT-SP1 was localized in the lumenal membrane of both normal and tumour prostate tissue, but a shedding of MT-SP1 into the lumen was only observed in a metastatic prostate cancer tissue sample. This soluble form of MT-SP1 might be suited as diagnostic marker for prostate cancer. Overall, highly specific and very potent HuCAL® antibody fragments against the cancer related human serine protease MT-SP1 were isolated directly from the HuCAL®-scFv library, without the need for further affinity engineering steps.

4.1.3   Application example: HuCAL® antibodies against FGFR3

Human fibroblast growth factor receptor 3 (FGFR3) belongs to a family of highly homologous cell surface expressed receptor tyrosine kinases (RTKs), which are involved in a multitude of cellular processes including cell growth, differentiation, migration, and survival (for review see Klint & Claesson-Welsh, 1999; Basilico & Moscatelli, 1992; Naski & Ornitz, 1998). Pathological disorders such as dwarfism or tumour genesis were linked to increased FGFR3 activity (for review see Webster & Donoghue, 1997; Burke *et al.*, 1998). The transforming potential of FGFR3 harbouring an activating mutation was shown for tumour progression of ectopically expressed FGFR3 in NIH3T3 cells and mouse bone marrow cells (Chesi *et al.*, 2001; Li *et al.*, 2001). Accordingly, high affinity human antibodies that block FGFR3 activity could be of great therapeutic benefit in treating FGFR3 mediated skeletal disorders and tumour genesis.

The HuCAL®-Fab 1 library was challenged with FGFR3 in a differential cell panning approach, performing three rounds of panning on immobilised recombinant protein alternating with cells expressing FGFR3 (Rauchenberger *et al.*, 2003). Several HuCAL®-Fab fragments were able to specifically inhibit FGFR3-mediated cell proliferation in the presence of the ligand FGF9. Some Fab fragments exhibit a monovalent affinity in the sub-nanomolar range and IC_{50} values below 20 nM. To our knowledge, these are the first monoclonal antibodies against FGFRs having functional blocking activity. The HuCAL®-Fab candidates will be further analysed in different *in vitro* and *in vivo* models to evaluate their therapeutic potential.

4.1.4   Application example: HuCAL® antibodies against ICAM-1

The intercellular adhesion molecule 1 (ICAM-1, CD54) is a member of the cell adhesion molecules that control interactions between leukocytes and vascular endothelial cells during an inflammatory reaction. ICAM-1 is expressed on endothelial cells and at moderate levels on a number of cells of the immune system, such as activated T- and B-lymphocytes and monocytes (Dustin *et al.*, 1986). Expression of ICAM-1 is strongly induced on endothelial cells by inflammatory cytokines such as interferon-gamma

(IFN-γ), interleukin-1 (IL-1) and tumour necrosis factor alpha (TNF-α) (Pober *et al.*, 1986). ICAM-1 plays a crucial role in inflammatory reactions mediating leukocyte extravasation by interacting with β2-integrins, mainly LFA-1 and Mac-1 on activated leukocytes (Marlin and Springer, 1987; Smith *et al.*, 1989; Diamond *et al.*, 1991). In addition, ICAM-1 functions as an accessory molecule on antigen presenting cells and delivers a co-stimulatory signal to T cells through interaction with LFA-1 (Dougherty *et al.*, 1988; Van Seventer *et al.*, 1990). As a key player in inflammation, ICAM-1 is a therapeutic target in diseases with inflammatory components, such as psoriasis and rheumatoid arthritis.

HuCAL® libraries were screened against ICAM-1, performing either three rounds of panning on immobilised recombinant antigen or alternating immobilised ICAM-1 with cells expressing ICAM-1. A range of antibodies were generated which specifically recognised ICAM-1 on cells, but had no cross-reactivity with the closely related ICAM-2 and ICAM-3 molecules. In total, four antibodies were characterised in great detail. Their monovalent affinities range from 3 nM to 80 nM, which after conversion into the IgG format translate to apparent K_D values of 1 to 3 nM. All HuCAL® antibodies are able to disrupt ICAM-1 mediated cell adhesion *in vitro,* as demonstrated in two settings. In a first assay, a completely cell-based system was applied analysing the monotypic aggregation of lymphoblastoid JY cells, which is dependent on the interaction of ICAM-1 and LFA-1 (Rothlein *et al.*, 1986). Second, the inhibitory potential of anti-ICAM-1 antibodies was quantified in a protein-cell adhesion assay which monitored the adhesion of LFA-1 expressing T-leukemia cells to immobilised recombinant ICAM-1. IC_{50} values as low as 3 nM were determined. In immunohistochemistry, all antibodies stained human tonsil tissue in a pattern expected for ICAM-1, demonstrating specific staining of endothelial cells around blood vessels and the reticular structure of germinal centres. Cross-reactivity with various non-human primates was shown for three antibodies, while one of them reacted also with mouse, rat and rabbit, facilitating *in vivo* studies in various animal models. Furthermore, specific IHC-staining of pathogenic tissues with elevated ICAM-1 levels could be demonstrated, such as endothelial cells and keratinocytes in skin tissue from psoriasis and burn patients. Further development of the antibodies in the indications psoriasis and deep dermal burn are ongoing.

4.2   Antibody Optimisation using HuCAL®

The examples described above prove that antibodies with therapeutic potential can be isolated directly from HuCAL® libraries without any engineering step. Their affinities are in the low nanomolar to even sub-nanomolar range. However, the unique design of HuCAL® in addition offers the option to further optimise selected antibodies with respect to affinity and specificity. The following section will describe the principles of HuCAL® antibody optimisation and will give an example by outlining the maturation of anti-HLA-DR antibodies.

4.2.1   Optimisation procedure

Phage display of diverse libraries of antibodies and other proteins has been extensively used to engineer molecules for improved affinity and specificity, applying a variety of different strategies (reviewed by Barbas & Burton, 1996; Rader & Barbas, 1997; Griffiths & Duncan, 1998). Methodologies, which direct modifications to the CDRs and leave the conserved germline-derived framework regions unchanged, have the great advantage of a reduced probability of generating immunogenic antibodies. Its unique modular structure renders HuCAL® the ideal basis for regio-specific optimisation of CDRs and gives rapid access to human antibodies with improved characteristics. The CDRs can easily be exchanged in a simple cloning step due to unique flanking restriction sites (Figure 2.6). Pre-built CDR cassette libraries are available ready-for-use. The consensus frameworks of HuCAL® antibodies are untouched in this process preserving the anticipated low immunogenicity of HuCAL® antibodies. By thorough analyses of the naturally occurring human CDR sequences, CDR libraries were constructed that mimic the CDRs of the natural human antibody repertoire, just as the six CDRs of HuCAL® GOLD do. These CDR libraries were constructed with MorphoSys' proprietary TRIM technology (see section 1.2), ensuring complete control over the amino acid composition and avoiding STOP codons. As a result, the CDR libraries are of substantially higher quality than using conventional mutagenesis approaches. Extensive quality control revealed more than 70 percent correct clones in the cassette libraries, resulting in a similar percentage of correct sequences after cloning of these cassettes into the parental Fab fragment.

This simple and efficient "*mix & match*"-process permits rapid affinity maturation of single HuCAL® antibodies ("lead optimisation") as well as entire pools of pre-selected HuCAL® antibodies ("pool optimisation"). To fully exploit the potential of this technology, we routinely apply a sequential optimisation of CDRs ("CDR walking", Yang *et al.*, 1995). Optimised binder(s) are used for the construction of a second library wherein a different CDR is diversified, and so on. Sequential optimisation takes into account that optimal binding may result from the interdependence of antigen binding by the different CDRs. The alternative approach is parallel optimisation, where different CDRs are optimised independently in parallel and later combined in one antibody fragment. The advantage of a parallel approach is clearly the speed to obtain the desired antibody. The obtained affinity improvement factors vary considerably and cannot be predicted beforehand (Yang *et al.*, 1995; Schier *et al.*, 1996a; Chen *et al.*, 1999). Overall, we have very good experience with both optimisation strategies obtaining antibodies with significantly improved affinities for all targets tested (examples given in Table 2.1).

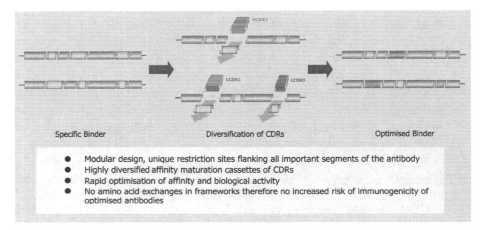

Figure 2.6. Antibody Optimisation using HuCAL®

Table 2.1. Examples of improvement factors and final monovalent affinities of HuCAL® antibody optimisation programs.

Parental Fab	Affinity improvement factor			Monovalent affinity [nM]
	1st round	2nd round	Combination of improved CDRs	
A	16	-*	-*	0.8
B	195	-*	-*	0.4
C	6	115	-*	3.0
D	16	1627	-*	0.03
E	2	9	14	0.5
F	29	69	3100	0.3

* - = not required

The generation of high affinity antibodies requires a stringent selection procedure. Various methods have been applied to increase stringency, including low antigen concentration, increased number of wash cycles, competition with excess of soluble antigen, competition with parental antibody fragments, and increased temperature (Hawkins *et al.*, 1992; Schier *et al.*, 1996a, b; Low *et al.*, 1996; Yang *et al.*, 1995; Chen *et al.*, 1999). The method of choice is dependent on i) the particular type and the available amount of antigen, ii) the applied panning procedure, and iii) the affinity of the parental antibody fragment. Due to the uncertainty regarding the highest affinity present in the diversified phage antibody library the optimal stringency conditions cannot be predicted *a priori*. Therefore on a regular basis, a range of different stringencies is applied in parallel. Alternatively, the optimisation protocol can be guided by determining the titre of eluted phages or the percentage of binding phages present in the phage eluate. Improvement factors in affinity of more than 3000-fold compared to the non-optimised parental antibodies could be shown, resulting in Fab fragments with monovalent sub-nanomolar to picomolar affinities. Table 2.1 summarizes some of the HuCAL® antibody optimisations. In all cases, high affinity antibodies were generated after up to two rounds of sequential or parallel optimisation. For example, one of them (Table 2.1, Fab F) showed exquisite biological functions but had a rather low monovalent affinity of 930 nM. In this case, optimisation resulted in a final binder with 3100-fold improved monovalent affinity of 300 pM and significantly increased biological activity. In another example, the parent Fab (Table 2.1, Fab A) already exhibited a good monovalent affinity of 13 nM. In just one round of maturation, the affinity was further improved by a factor of 16 reaching 800 pM in the Fab format. It could be shown that the increased affinity correlated with improved efficacy: IC_{50} values were 11 nM for the parental Fab, and about 1 nM after optimisation. In the following section the optimisation of anti-HLA-DR antibodies is described in more detail.

4.2.2   Application example: Optimisation of anti-HLA-DR antibodies

Anti-MHC II antibodies are of great value as therapeutic agents for the treatment of lymphoma/leukemia. Several MHC-II specific murine monoclonal antibodies have been shown to induce programmed death of MHC class II positive tumour cells (Vaickus *et al.*, 1989; Newell *et al.*, 1993; Truman *et al.*, 1994; Vidovic & Toral, 1998), and demonstrated efficacy and specific tumour killing in *in vivo* mouse lymphoma models (Bridges *et al.*, 1987). In order to generate fully human antibodies with similar biological activity, HuCAL® was screened against the human leukocyte antigen-DR (HLA-DR) (Nagy *et al.*, 2002). A protein solid-phase panning with purified HLA-DR molecules was performed as well as a differential cell panning with purified HLA-DR molecules and cells expressing HLA-DR. Twelve specific antibody fragments were obtained, four of which exhibited strong tumour killing activity, when dimerised via cross-linking with an antibody directed against a specific tag at the Fab. The monovalent fragments were not tumouricidal, confirming earlier observations by Vidovic *et al.* (1995). Four antibodies with the desired biological activity had modest affinities and were subjected to two sequential rounds of affinity maturation. In the first round of optimisation, the L-CDR3-sequences were diversified. The four libraries (one for each selected antibody) were kept separate and were subjected to either two rounds of standard solid-phase-panning, or one round of solid-phase panning on purified HLA-DR molecules followed by whole-cell panning on cells expressing HLA-DR. The best Fab candidate was improved by a factor of six compared to its parental Fab reaching a monovalent K_D of 59 nM. In the second round of affinity maturation, optimisation of L-CDR1 was performed. Prolonged wash cycles and addition of competing antigen led to the selection of several Fab fragments with affinities in the range of 3 nM. Finally, the best candidates were converted into IgG4 antibodies exhibiting sub-nanomolar functional affinities while preserving specificity. The optimised anti-HLA-DR antibody has potent killing activity against a series of lymphoma and leukemia cell lines and against samples from chronic lymphocytic leukemia patients *in vitro*, while normal resting lymphocytes are not affected. Cell death occurs without the need for additional immunological effector mechanisms or toxin conjugation. In addition, *in vivo* efficacy could be shown in animal models of non-Hodgkin's lymphoma, Hodgkin's lymphoma, multiple myeloma, and hairy cell leukemia (Nagy *et al.*, 2002; www.gpc-ag.com).

5.   SUMMARY

This article describes the Human Combinatorial Antibody Library (HuCAL®) technology and demonstrates its versatility for target research and therapeutic applications. HuCAL® offers the advantages to generate a variety of highly specific and fully human monoclonal antibodies against any antigen of choice, even toxic or conserved ones. Since it is an *in vitro* technology, based on phage display, selection conditions can be adjusted at will. The antigen can be presented as isolated molecule or on the surface of cells, and automated high-throughput procedures for antibody generation and production have been set up (AutoCAL™). The modular design of the HuCAL® antibody genes and expression vectors allows the straightforward conversion of selected antibodies into various formats and isotypes, without changing the parental sequences. If required, systematic and rapid antibody engineering facilitates further antibody optimisation. This process is restricted to the CDRs, while the consensus frameworks, which are very close or even identical to human germline sequences remain untouched. HuCAL® technologies not only provide the method of choice for antibody generation facilitated by the novel CysDisplay™ technology, they also offer the high-throughput production of EST-encoded polypeptides (HuCAL®-EST) serving as antigens. Moreover, for the selection of the lead antibody candidates, efficient screening and validation methods have been established, such as high-throughput affinity ranking, immunohistochemistry and a variety of functional assays. HuCAL® therefore facilitates a seamless transition from target validation and drug discovery to the development of therapeutic antibodies.

ACKNOWLEDGEMENT

The authors would like to thank the entire team at MorphoSys for their excellent work in the projects described above, Titus Kretzschmar for stimulating discussions and Sabine Brettreich for preparation of the manuscript. MorphoSys greatly appreciates the financial support given by the *Bundesministerium für Bildung und Forschung* (BMBF) and the *Bayerische Forschungsstiftung* (BFS) for some of the projects.

REFERENCES

Adams, M. D., Kerlavage, A. R., Fleischmann, R. D., Fuldner, R. A., Bult, C. J., Lee, N. H., Kirkness, E. F., Weinstock, K. G., Gocayne, J. D. and White, O., 1995, Initial assessment of human gene diversity and expression patterns based upon 83 million nucleotides of cDNA sequence. *Nature* 377 (6547 Suppl): 3-174.

Bachelez, H., Flageul, B., Dubertret, L., Fraitag, S., Grossman, R., Brousse, N., Poisson, D., Knowles, R.W., Wacholtz, M.C., Haverty, T.P., Chatenoud, L., and Bach, J.F., 1998, Treatment of recalcitrant plaque psoriasis with a humanized non-depleting antibody to CD4. *J. Autoimmun.* 11: 53-62.

Baker, K.N., Rendall, M.H., Hills, A.E., Hoare, M., Freedman, R.B., and James, D.C., 2001, Metabolic control of recombinant protein N-glycan processing in NS0 and CHO cells. *Biotechnol. Bioeng.* 73: 188-202.

Bakker, H., Bardor, M., Molthoff, J.W., Gomord, V., Elbers, I., Stevens, L.H., Jordi, W., Lommen, A., Faye, L., Lerouge, P., and Bosch, D., 2001, Galactose-extended glycans of antibodies produced by transgenic plants. *Proc. Natl. Acad. Sci. USA* 98: 2899-2904.

Barbas, C.F. III. and Burton, D.R., 1996, Selection and evolution of high-affinity human anti-viral antibodies. *Trends Biotechnol.* 14: 230-234

Basilico, C. and Moscatelli, D., 1992, The FGF family of growth factors and oncogenes. *Adv. Cancer Res.* 59: 115-165

Better, M., Chang, C.P., Robinson, R.R., and Horwitz, A.H., 1988, *Escherichia coli* secretion of an active chimeric antibody fragment. *Science,* 240: 1041-1043.

Boder, E. T. and Wittrup, K. D., 2000, Yeast surface display for directed evolution of protein expression, affinity, and stability. *Methods Enzymol.* 328:430-444.

Bothmann, H. and Plückthun, A., 1998, Selection for a periplasmic factor improving phage display and functional periplasmic expression. *Nat. Biotechnol.* 16: 376-380.

Brandts, J.F., Hu, C.Q., Lin, L.N., and Mos, M.T., 1989, A simple model for proteins with interacting domains. Applications to scanning calorimetry data. *Biochemistry*, **28**: 8588-8596.

Breedveld, F.C., 2000, Therapeutic monoclonal antibodies. *Lancet*, **355**: 735-740.

Bridges, S.H., Kruisbeek, A.M., and Longo, D.L., 1987, Selective *in vivo* antitumour effects of monoclonal anti-I-A antibody on B cell lymphoma. *J. Immunol.* **139**: 4242-4249

Buchner, J. and Rudolph, R., 1991, Renaturation, purification and characterization of recombinant Fab-fragments produced in *Escherichia coli*. *Biotechnology (N. Y.)*, **9**: 157-162.

Burke, D., Wilkes, D., Blundell, T.L., and Malcolm, S., 1998, Fibroblast growth factor receptors: lessons from the genes. *Trends Biochem. Sci.* **23**: 59-62

Cahill, D.J., 2001, Protein and antibody arrays and their medical applications. *J. Immunol. Methods*, **250**: 81-91.

Carayannopoulos, L., Max, E.E., and Capra, J.D., 1994, Recombinant human IgA expressed in insect cells. *Proc. Natl. Acad. Sci. U. S. A*, **91**: 8348-8352.

Carter, P., 2001, Bispecific human IgG by design. *J. Immunol. Methods*, **248**: 7-15.

Chapman, A.P., Antoniw, P., Spitali, M., West, S., Stephens, S., and King, D.J., 1999, Therapeutic antibody fragments with prolonged *in vivo* half-lives. *Nat. Biotechnol.*, **17**: 780-783.

Chapman, A.P., 2002, PEGylated antibodies and antibody fragments for improved therapy: a review. *Adv. Drug Deliv. Rev.*, **54**: 531-545.

Chen, W., and Georgiou, G., 2002, Cell-surface display of heterologous proteins: From high-throughput screening to environmental applications. *Biotechnol. Bioeng.* **79**:496-503.

Chen, Y., Wiesmann, C., Fuh, G., Li, B., Christinger, H.W., McKay, P., de Vos, A.M., and Lowman, H.B., 1999, Selection and analysis of an optimised anti-VEGF antibody: Crystal structure of an affinity-matured Fab in complex with antigen. *J. Mol. Biol.* **293**: 865-881

Chesi, M., Brents, L.A., Ely, S.A., Bais, C., Robbiani, D.F., Mesri, E.A., Kuehl, W.M., and Bergsagel, P.L., 2001, Activated fibroblast growth factor receptor 3 is an oncogene that contributes to tumour progression in multiple myeloma. *Blood* **97**: 729-736

Cho, M.S., Yee, H., Brown, C., Mei, B., Mirenda, C., and Chan, S., 2003, Versatile expression system for rapid and stable production of recombinant proteins. *Biotechnol. Prog.*, **19**: 229-232.

Choy, E.H., Hazleman, B., Smith, M., Moss, K., Lisi, L., Scott, D.G., Patel, J., Sopwith, M., and Isenberg, D.A., 2002, Efficacy of a novel PEGylated humanized anti-TNF fragment (CDP870) in patients with rheumatoid arthritis: a phase II double-blinded, randomized, dose-escalating trial. *Rheumatology (Oxford)*, **41**: 1133-1137.

Davis, T.A., Grillo-Lopez, A.J., White, C.A., McLaughlin, P., Czuczman, M.S., Link, B.K., Maloney, D.G., Weaver, R.L., Rosenberg, J., and Levy, R., 2000, Rituximab anti-CD20 monoclonal antibody therapy in non-Hodgkin's lymphoma: safety and efficacy of re-treatment. *J. Clin. Oncol.*, **18**: 3135-3143.

de Haard, H. J., van Neer, N., Reurs, A., Hufton, S. E., Roovers, R. C., Henderikx, P., de Bruine, A. P., Arends, J.-W. and Hoogenboom, H., 1999, A large non-immunized human Fab fragment phage library that permits rapid isolation and kinetic analysis of high affinity antibodies. *J. Biol. Chem.* **274**: 18218 – 18230.

de Wildt, R.M., Mundy, C.R., Gorick, B.D., and Tomlinson, I.M., 2000, Antibody arrays for high-throughput screening of antibody-antigen interactions. *Nat. Biotechnol.* **18**: 989-994.

Diamond, M.S., Staunton, D.E., Marlin, S.D., and Springer, T.A., 1991, Binding of the integrin Mac-1 (CD11b/CD18) to the third immunoglobulin-like domain of ICAM-1 (CD54) and its regulation by glycosylation. *Cell* **65**: 961-971

Dougherty, G.J., Murdoch, S., and Hogg, N., 1988, The function of human intercellular adhesion molecule-1 (ICAM-1) in the generation of an immune response. *Eur. J. Immunol.* 18: 35-39

Dreier, T., Lorenczewski, G., Brandl, C., Hoffmann, P., Syring, U., Hanakam, F., Kufer, P., Riethmüller, G., Bargou, R., Baeuerle, P. A., 2002, Extremely potent, rapid and costimulation-independent cytotoxic T-cell response against lymphoma cells catalysed by a single chain bispecific antibody. *Int. J. Cancer* 100: 690-697.

Dustin, M.L., Rothlein, R., Bhan, A.K., Dinarello, C.A., and Springer, T.A., 1986, Induction by IL 1 and interferon-gamma: tissue distribution, biochemistry, and function of a natural adherence molecule (ICAM-1). *J. Immunol.* 137: 245-254

Eickhoff, H., Konthur, Z., Lueking, A., Lehrach, H., Walter, G., Nordhoff, E., Nyarsik, L. and Bussow,K., 2002, Protein array technology: the tool to bridge genomics and proteomics. *Adv. Biochem. Eng. Biotechnol.* 77: 103-112.

Ewert, S., Honegger, A. and Plückthun, A., 2003b, Structure-based improvement of the biophysical properties of immunoglobulin v(h) domains with a generalizable approach. *Biochemistry*, 42: 1517-1528.

Ewert, S., Huber, T., Honegger, A. and Plückthun, A., 2003a, Biophysical properties of human antibody variable domains. *J. Mol. Biol.* 325: 531-553.

Forsberg, G., Forsgren, M., Jaki, M., Norin, M., Sterky, C., Enhorning, A., Larsson, K., Ericsson, M. and Bjork, P., 1997, Identification of framework residues in a secreted recombinant antibody fragment that control production level and localization in *Escherichia coli. J. Biol. Chem.* 272: 12430-12436.

Frisch, C., Brocks, B., Ostendorp, R., Hoess, A., von Rüden, T. and Kretzschmar, T., 2003, From EST to IHC: human antibody pipeline for target research. *J. Immunol. Methods* 275: 203-212.

Gessner, J.E., Heiken H., Tamm,A., and Schmidt,R.E., 1998, The IgG Fc receptor family. *Ann. Hematol.* 76: 231-248.

Glennie, M. J. and Johnson, P. W. M., 2000, Clinical trials of antibody therapy. *Immunol. Today* 21: 403-410.

Griffiths, A. D., Williams, S. C., Hartley, O., Tomlinson, I. M., Waterhouse, P., Crosby, W. L., Kontermann, R. E., Jones, P. T., Low, N. M., Allison, T. J., Prospero, T. D., Hoogenboom, H. R., Nissim, A., Cox, J. P. L., Harrison, J. L., Zaccolo, M., Gherardi, E. and Winter, G., 1994, Isolation of high affinity human antibodies directly from large synthetic repertoires. *EMBO J.* 13: 3245 – 3260.

Griffiths, A.D. and Duncan, A.R., 1998, Strategies for selection of antibodies by phage display. *Curr. Opin. Biotechnol.* 9: 102-108.

Grillo-Lopez, A.J., 2002, Zevalin: the first radioimmunotherapy approved for the treatment of lymphoma. *Expert Rev. Anticancer Ther.* 2: 485-493.

Gumpert, J. and Hoischen, C., 1998, Use of cell wall-less bacteria (L-forms) for efficient expression and secretion of heterologous gene products. *Curr. Opin. Biotechnol.* 9: 506-509.

Gura, T. 2002, Therapeutic antibodies: magic bullets hit the target. *Nature* 417: 584-586.

Haab, B.B., Dunham, M.J., and Brown, P.O., 2001, Protein microarrays for highly parallel detection and quantitation of specific proteins and antibodies in complex solutions. *Genome Biol.* 2: RESEARCH0004.

Hanes, J., Jermutus, L. and Plückthun, A., 2000, Selecting and evolving functional proteins *in vitro* by ribosome display. *Methods Enzymol.* 328: 404-430.

Harris, J.L. and Craik, C.S., 2000, Proteases: The tip of the iceberg. *Cell* 101: 136-137.

Hawkins, R.E., Russell, S.J. and Winter, G., 1992, Selection of phage antibodies by binding affinity. Mimicking affinity maturation. *J. Mol. Biol.* 226: 889-896.

Hayhurst, A. and Georgiou, G., 2001, High-throughput antibody isolation. *Curr. Opin. Chem. Biol.* **5**: 683-689.

Hiniker, A. and Bardwell, J.C., 2003, Disulfide bond isomerisation in prokaryotes. *Biochemistry* **42**: 1179-1185.

Holliger, P., Prospero, T. and Winter, G., 1993, "Diabodies": Small bivalent and bispecific antibody fragments. *Proc. Natl. Acad. Sci. USA* **90**: 6444-6448.

Holliger, P. and Hoogenboom, H., 1998, Antibodies come back from the brink. *Nat Biotechnol,* **16**: 1015-1016.

Hoogenboom, H.R., Lutgerink, J.T., Pelsers, M.M., Rousch, M.J., Coote, J., van Neer, N., de Bruine, A., van Nieuwenhoven, F.A., Glatz, J.F., and Arends, J.W., 1999, Selection-dominant and nonaccessible epitopes on cell-surface receptors revealed by cell-panning with a large phage antibody library. *Eur. J. Biochem.* **260**: 774-784.

Hooper, J.D., Clements, J.A., Quigley, J.P., and Antails, T.M., 2001, Type II transmembrane serine protease. *J. Biol. Chem.* **276**: 857-860.

Horn, U., Strittmatter, W., Krebber, A., Knupfer, U., Kujau, M., Wenderoth, R., Muller, K., Matzku, S., Plückthun, A., and Riesenberg, D., 1996, High volumetric yields of functional dimeric miniantibodies in *Escherichia coli*, using an optimised expression vector and high-cell-density fermentation under non-limited growth conditions. *Appl. Microbiol. Biotechnol.* **46**: 524-532.

Huls, G.A., Heijnen, I.A., Cuomo, M.E., Koningsberger, J.C., Wiegman, L., Boel, E., van der Vuurst de Vries, A.R., Loyson, S.A., Helfrich, W., van Berge Henegouwen , G.P., van Meijer, M., De Kruif, J. and Logtenberg, T., 1999, A recombinant, fully human monoclonal antibody with anti-tumour activity constructed from phage-displayed antibody fragments. *Nature Biotech.* **17**: 276-281.

Humphreys, D.P., Chapman, A.P., Reeks, D.G., Lang, V. and Stephens, P.E., 1997, Formation of dimeric Fabs in *Escherichia coli*: effect of hinge size and isotype, presence of interchain disulphide bond, Fab' expression levels, tail piece sequences and growth conditions. *J. Immunol. Methods* **209**: 193-202.

Humphreys, D.P., Vetterlein, O.M., Chapman, A.P., King, D.J., Antoniw, P., Suitters, A.J., Reeks, D.G., Parton, T.A., King, L.M., Smith, B.J., Lang, V. and Stephens, P.E., 1998, F(ab')2 molecules made from *Escherichia coli* produced Fab' with hinge sequences conferring increased serum survival in an animal model. *J. Immunol. Methods* **217**: 1-10.

Humphreys, D.P. and Glover, D.J., 2001, Therapeutic antibody production technologies: molecules, applications, expression and purification. *Curr. Opin. Drug Discov. Devel.* **4**: 172-185.

Humphreys, D.P., Carrington, B., Bowering, L.C., Ganesh, R., Sehdev, M., Smith, B.J., King, L.M., Reeks, D.G., Lawson, A. and Popplewell, A.G., 2002, A plasmid system for optimisation of Fab(') production in *Escherichia coli*: importance of balance of heavy chain and light chain synthesis. *Protein Expr. Purif.,* **26**: 309-320.

Jaenicke, R. and Lilie, H., 2000, Folding and association of oligomeric and multimeric proteins. *Adv. Protein Chem.* **53**: 329-401.

Jaenicke, R., Schurig, H., Beaucamp, N. and Ostendorp, R., 1996, Structure and stability of hyperstable proteins: glycolytic enzymes from the hyperthermophilic bacterium *Thermotoga maritima. Adv. Protein Chem.* **48**: 181-269.

Jaffers, G., Fuller, T. C., Cosimi, A. B., Russell, P. S., Winn, H. J. and Colvin, R. B., 1986, Monoclonal antibody therapy. Anti-idiotypic and non-anti-idiotypic antibodies to OKT3 arising despite intense immunosuppression. *Transplantation* **41**: 572 – 578.

Jefferis, R., Lund, J., and Pound, J.D., 1998, IgG-Fc-mediated effector functions: molecular definition of interaction sites for effector ligands and the role of glycosylation. *Immunol. Rev.* **163**: 59-76.

Jefferis, R. and Lund, J., 2002, Interaction sites on human IgG-Fc for FcgammaR: current models. *Immunol. Lett.*, **82**: 57-65.

Jermutus, L., Ryabova, L.A. and Plückthun, A., 1998, Recent advances in producing and selecting functional proteins by using cell-free translation. *Curr. Opin. Biotechnol.* **9**: 534-548.

Jiang, X., Ookubo, Y., Fujii, I., Nakano, H. and Yamane, T., 2002, Expression of Fab fragment of catalytic antibody 6D9 in an *Escherichia coli in vitro* coupled transcription/translation system. *FEBS Lett.* **514**: 290-294.

Jirholt, P., Ohlin, M., Borrebaeck, C. A. K. and Söderlind, E., 1998, Exploiting sequence space: shuffling *in vivo* formed complementarity determining regions into a master framework. *Gene* **215**: 471 – 476.

Jones, D., Kroos, N., Anema, R., Van Montfort, B., Vooys, A., Van Der, K.S., Van Der, H.E., Smits, S., Schouten, J., Brouwer, K., Lagerwerf, F., Van Berkel, P., Opstelten, D.J., Logtenberg, T. and Bout, A., 2003, High-level expression of recombinant IgG in the human cell line per.c6. *Biotechnol. Prog.* **19**: 163-168.

Joos, T. O., Stoll, D., Templin, M., Virnekäs, B., and Ostendorp, R., 2002, Method for the relative determination of physicochemical properties. WO 02/086494.

Joos, T.O., Stoll, D. and Templin, M.F., 2002, Miniaturised multiplexed immunoassays. *Curr. Opin. Chem. Biol.* **6**: 76-80.

Kellermann, S. A. and Green, L. L., 2002, Antibody discovery: the use of transgenic mice to generate human monoclonal antibodies for therapeutics. *Curr. Opin. Biotechnol.* **13**:593-597.

Kigawa, T., Yabuki, T., Yoshida, Y., Tsutsui, M., Ito, Y., Shibata, T. and Yokoyama, S., 1999, Cell-free production and stable-isotope labeling of milligram quantities of proteins. *FEBS Lett.* **442**: 15-19.

King, A., Boocock, C., Sharkey, A.M., Gardner, L., Beretta, A., Siccardi, A.G. and Loke, Y.W., 1996a, Evidence for the expression of HLA-C class I mRNA and protein by human first trimester trophoblast. *J. Immunol.* **156**: 2068-2076.

King, A., Burrows, T., and Locke, Y.W., 1996b, Human uterine natural killer cells. *Nat. Immun.* **15**: 41-52.

Kipriyanov, S.M., Moldenhauer, G., Schuhmacher, J., Cochlovius, B., der Lieth, C.W., Matys, E.R., and Little, M., 1999, Bispecific tandem diabody for tumour therapy with improved antigen binding and pharmacokinetics. *J Mol Biol*, **293**: 41-56.

Klint, P. and Claesson-Welsh, L., 1999, Signal transduction by fibroblast growth factor receptors. *Front. Biosci.* **4**: D165-177.

Knappik, A., Ge, L., Honegger, A., Pack, P., Fischer, M., Wellnhofer, G., Hoess, A., Wölle, J., Plückthun, A. and Virnekäs, B., 2000, Fully synthetic Human Combinatorial Antibody Libraries (HuCAL) based on modular consensus frameworks and CDRs randomized with trinucleotides. *J. Mol. Biol.* **296**: 57-86.

Köhler, G. and Milstein, C., 1975, Continuous cultures of fused cells secreting antibody of predefined specificity. *Nature* **256**: 495-497.

Krebs, B., Rauchenberger, R., Reiffert, S., Rothe, C., Tesar, M., Thomassen, E., Cao, M., Dreier, T., Fischer, D., Höß, A., Inge, L., Knappik, A., Marget, M., Pack, P., Meng, X., Schier, R., Söhlemann, P., Winter, J., Wölle, J. and Kretzschmar, T., 2001, High-throughput generation and engineering of recombinant human antibodies. *J. Immunol. Methods* **254**: 67-84.

Kretzschmar, T. and von Rüden, T., 2002, Antibody discovery: phage display. *Curr. Opin. Biotechnol.* **13**: 598-602.

Kujau, M.J., Hoischen, C., Riesenberg, D. and Gumpert, J., 1998, Expression and secretion of functional miniantibodies McPC603scFvDhlx in cell-wall-less L-form strains of *Proteus mirabilis* and *Escherichia coli*: a comparison of the synthesis capacities of L-form strains with an *E. coli* producer strain. *Appl. Microbiol. Biotechnol.* **49**: 51-58.

Laden, J.C., Philibert, P., Torreilles, F., Pugniere, M. and Martineau, P., 2002, Expression and folding of an antibody fragment selected *in vivo* for high expression levels in *Escherichia coli* cytoplasm. *Res. Microbiol.* **153**: 469-474.

Lesley, S.A., 2001, High-throughput proteomics: protein expression and purification in the postgenomic world. *Protein Expr. Purif.* **22**: 159-164.

Li, Z., Zhu, Y.X., Plowright, E.E., Bergsagel, P.L., Chesi, M., Patterson, B., Hawley, T.S., Hawley, R.G., and Stewart, A.K., 2001, The myeloma-associated oncogene fibroblast growth factor receptor 3 is transforming in hematopoietic cells. *Blood* **97**: 2413-2419.

Lilie, H., Lang, K., Rudolph, R. and Buchner, J., 1993, Prolyl isomerases catalyze antibody folding *in vitro*. *Protein Sci.* **2**: 1490-1496.

Lin, C.Y., Anders, J., Johnson, M. and Dickson, R.B., 1999a, Purification and characterization of a complex containing matriptase and a Kunitz-type serine protease inhibitor from human milk. *J. Biol. Chem.* **274**: 18237-18242.

Lin, C.Y., Anders, J., Johnson, M., Sang, Q.A., and Dickson, R.B., 1999b, Molecular cloning of cDNA for matriptase, a matrix-degrading serine protease with trypsin-like activity. *J. Biol. Chem.* **274**: 18231-18236.

Little, M., Kipriyanov, S. M., Le Gall, F. and Moldenhauer, G., 2000, Of mice and men: hybridoma and recombinant antibodies. *Immunol. Today* **21**: 364-370.

Löhning, C., 2001, Novel methods for displaying (poly)peptides/proteins on bacteriophage particles via disulfide bonds. WO 01/05950.

Lorenz, H.M., 2002, Technology evaluation: adalimumab, Abbott laboratories. *Curr. Opin. Mol. Ther.* **4**: 185-190.

Low, N.M., Holliger, P. and Winter, G., 1996, Mimicking somatic hypermutation: affinity maturation of antibodies displayed on bacteriophage using a bacterial mutator strain. *J. Mol. Biol.* **260**: 359-368.

Lu,D., Jimenez,X., Zhang,H., Bohlen,P., Witte,L., and Zhu,Z., 2002, Fab-scFv fusion protein: an efficient approach to production of bispecific antibody fragments. *J Immunol Methods,* **267**: 213-226.

Lueking, A., Horn, M., Eickhoff, H., Bussow, K., Lehrach, H. and Walter, G., 1999, Protein microarrays for gene expression and antibody screening. *Anal. Biochem.* **270**: 103-111.

MacBeath, G. and Schreiber, S.L., 2000, Printing proteins as microarrays for high-throughput function determination. *Science* **289**: 1760-1763.

Marget, M., Sharma, B.B., Tesar, M., Kretzschmar, T., Jenisch, S., Westphal, E., Davarnia, P., Weiss, E., Ulbrecht, M., Kabelitz, D. and Krönke, M., 2000, Bypassing hybridoma technology: HLA-C reactive human single-chain antibody fragments (scFv) derived from a synthetic phage display library (HuCAL) and their potential to discriminate HLA class I specificities. *Tissue Antigens* **56**: 1–9.

Marlin, S.D. and Springer, T.A., 1987, Purified intercellular adhesion molecule-1 (ICAM-1) is a ligand for lymphocyte function-associated antigen 1 (LFA-1). *Cell* **51**: 813-819.

Martineau, P., Jones, P. and Winter, G., 1998, Expression of an antibody fragment at high levels in the bacterial cytoplasm. *J. Mol. Biol.* **280**: 117-127.

Matthews, B.W., 1995, Studies on protein stability with T4 lysozyme. *Adv. Protein Chem.,* **46**: 249-278.

Milstein, C. and Cuello, A.C., 1983, Hybrid hybridomas and their use in immunohistochemistry. *Nature* **305**: 537-540.

Mimura, Y., Ghirlando, R., Sondermann, P., Lund, J. and Jefferis, R., 2001, The molecular specificity of IgG-Fc interactions with Fc gamma receptors. *Adv. Exp. Med. Biol.* **495**: 49-53.

Morton, H.C., Atkin, J.D., Owens, R.J. and Woof, J.M., 1993, Purification and characterization of chimeric human IgA1 and IgA2 expressed in COS and Chinese hamster ovary cells. *J. Immunol.* **151**: 4743-4752.

Mourad, G.J., Preffer, F.I., Wee, S.L., Powelson, J.A., Kawai, T., Delmonico, F.L., Knowles, R.W., Cosimi, A.B. and Colvin, R.B., 1998, Humanized IgG1 and IgG4 anti-CD4 monoclonal antibodies: effects on lymphocytes in the blood, lymph nodes, and renal allografts in *cynomolgus* monkeys. *Transplantation*, **65**: 632-641.

Nagy, Z. A., Hubner, B., Löhning, C., Rauchenberger, R., Reiffert, S., Thomassen-Wolf, E., Zahn, S., Leyer, S., Schier, E. M., Zahradnik, A., Brunner, C., Stanglmaier, M., Anderson, S., Dunn, M., Hallek, M., Kretzschmar, T. and Tesar, M., 2002, Fully human, HLA-DR-specific monoclonal antibodies efficiently induce programmed death of malignant lymphoid cells. *Nat. Med.* **8**: 801-807.

Naski, M.C. and Ornitz, D.M., 1998, FGF signaling in skeletal development. *Front. Biosci.* **3**: D781-794.

Newell, M.K., VanderWall, J., Beard, K.S. and Freed, J.H., 1993, Ligation of major histocompatiblity complex class II molecules mediates apoptotic cell death in resting B lymphocytes. *Proc. Natl. Acad. Sci. USA* **90**: 10459-10463.

O'Shea, E.K., Rutkowski, R., Stafford, W.F.III and Kim, P.S., 1989, Preferential heterodimer formation by isolated leucine zippers from fos and jun. *Science* **245**: 646-648.

Pack, P. and Plückthun, A., 1992, Miniantibodies: use of amphipathic helices to produce functional, flexibly linked dimeric Fv fragments with high avidity in *Escherichia coli*. *Biochemistry* **31**: 1579-1584.

Pack, P., Kujau, M., Schroeckh, V., Knupfer, U., Wenderoth, R., Riesenberg, D. and Plückthun, A., 1993, Improved bivalent miniantibodies, with identical avidity as whole antibodies, produced by high cell density fermentation of *Escherichia coli*. *Biotechnology (N. Y.)* **11**: 1271-1277.

Pack, P., Muller, K., Zahn, R. and Plückthun, A., 1995, Tetravalent miniantibodies with high avidity assembling in *Escherichia coli*. *J. Mol. Biol.* **246**: 28-34.

Palomares, L.A., Joosten, C.E., Hughes, P.R., Granados, R.R. and Shuler, M.L., 2003, Novel insect cell line capable of complex N-glycosylation and sialylation of recombinant proteins. *Biotechnol. Prog.* **19**: 185-192.

Peluso, P., Wilson, D.S., Do, D., Tran, H., Venkatasubbaiah, M., Quincy, D., Heidecker, B., Poindexter, K., Tolani, N., Phelan, M., Witte, K., Jung, L.S., Wagner, P. and Nock, S., 2003, Optimising antibody immobilization strategies for the construction of protein microarrays. *Anal. Biochem.* **312**: 113-124.

Perelson, A. S., 1989, Immune network theory. *Immunol. Rev.* **110**: 5 – 36.

Persic, L., Horn, I. R., Rybak, S., Cattaneo, A., Hoogenboom, H. R. and Bradbury, A., 1999, Single-chain variable fragments selected on the 57-76 p21Ras neutralising epitope from phage antibody libraries recognise the parental protein. *FEBS Lett.* **443**:112-116.

Plückthun, A., Krebber, A., Krebber, C., Horn, U., Knüpfer, U., Wenderoth, R., Nieba, L., Proba, K. and Riesenberg, D., 1996, Producing antibodies in *Escherichia coli*: from PCR to fermentation. *In*: B.D. Hames (ed.), Antibody Engineering, pp. 203-249. Oxford, United Kingdom: Oxford University Press.

Plückthun, A. and Pack, P., 1997, New protein engineering approaches to multivalent and bispecific antibody fragments. *Immunotechnology* **3**: 83-105.

Pober, J.S., Gimbrone, M.A.Jr, Lapierre, L.A., Mendrick, D.L., Fiers, W., Rothlein, R., and Springer T.A., 1986, Overlapping patterns of activation of human endothelial cells by interleukin 1, tumour necrosis factor, and immune interferon. *J. Immunol.* **137**: 1893-1896.

Queen, C., Schneider, W. P., Selick, H. E., Payne, P. W., Landolfi, N. F., Duncan, J. F., Avdalovic, N. M., Levitt, M., Junghans, R. P. and Waldmann, T. A., 1989, A humanized antibody that binds to the interleukin 2 receptor. *Proc. Natl. Acad. Sci. USA* **86**: 10029-10033.

Rader, C. and Barbas, C.F.III., 1997, Phage display of combinatorial antibody libraries. *Curr. Opin. Biotechnol.* **8**: 503-508.

Ramjiawan, B., Maiti, P., Aftanas, A., Kaplan, H., Fast, D., Mantsch, H.H. and Jackson, M., 2000, Noninvasive localization of tumours by immunofluorescence imaging using a single chain Fv fragment of a human monoclonal antibody with broad cancer specificity. *Cancer* **89**:1134-1144.

Rauchenberger, R., Borges, E., Thomassen-Wolf, E., Rom, E., Adar, R., Vaniv, Y., Malka, A., Cumakov, I., Kotzer, S., Resnitzky, D., Knappik, A., Reiffert, S., Prassler, J., Jury, K., Waldherr, D., Bauer, S., Kretzschmar, T., Yayon, A. and Rothe, C., Human combinatorial Fab library, HuCAL®-Fab 1, yielding the first specific and functional antibodies against the human receptor tyrosine kinase FGFR3. *J. Biol. Chem.* 2003, In press

Reichert, J.M., 2001, Monoclonal antibodies in the clinic. *Nat. Biotechnol.* **19**: 819-822.

Reichert, J.M., 2002, Therapeutic monoclonal antibodies: trends in development and approval in the US. *Curr. Opin. Mol. Ther.* **4**: 110-118.

Rheinnecker, M., Hardt, C., Ilag, L.L., Kufer, P., Gruber, R., Hoess, A., Lupas, A., Rottenberger, C., Plückthun, A. and Pack, P., 1996, Multivalent antibody fragments with high functional affinity for a tumour-associated carbohydrate antigen. *J. Immunol.* **157**: 2989-2997.

Rippmann, J.F., Klein, M., Hoischen, C., Brocks, B., Rettig, W.J., Gumpert, J., Pfizenmaier, K., Mattes, R. and Moosmayer, D., 1998, Procaryotic expression of single-chain variable-fragment (scFv) antibodies: secretion in L-form cells of *Proteus mirabilis* leads to active product and overcomes the limitations of periplasmic expression in *Escherichia coli. Appl. Environ. Microbiol.* **64**: 4862-4869.

Rothlein, R., Dustin, M.L., Marlin, S.D. and Springer, T.A., 1986, A human intercellular adhesion molecule (ICAM-1) distinct from LFA-1. *J. Immunol.* **137**: 1270-1274.

Ryabova, L.A., Desplancq, D., Spirin, A.S. and Plückthun, A., 1997, Functional antibody production using cell-free translation: effects of protein disulfide isomerase and chaperones. *Nat. Biotechnol.* **15**: 79-84.

Sblattero, D. and Bradbury, A., 2000, Exploiting recombination in single bacteria to make large phage antibody libraries. *Nat. Biotech.* **18**: 75 – 80.

Schäffner, J., Winter, J., Rudolph, R. and Schwarz, E., 2001, Cosecretion of chaperones and low-molecular-size medium additives increases the yield of recombinant disulfide-bridged proteins. *Appl. Environ. Microbiol.* **67**: 3994-4000.

Schellekens, H., 2002, Immunogenicity of therapeutic proteins: clinical implications and future prospects. *Clin Ther.* **24**: 1720-1740.

Schier, R., Bye, J., Apell, G., Mc Call, A., Adams, G.P., Malmqvist, M., Weiner, L.M. and Marks, J.D., 1996a, Isolation of high-affinity monomeric human anti-c-erbB2 single chain Fv using affinity-driven selection. *J. Mol. Biol.* **255**: 28-43.

Schier, R., McCall, A., Adams, G.P., Marshall, K.W., Merritt, H., Yim, M., Crawford, R.S., Weiner, L.M., Marks, C. and Marks, J.D., 1996b, Isolation of picomolar affinity anti-c-erbB-2 single-chain Fv by molecular evolution of the complementarity determining regions in the center of the antibody binding site. *J. Mol. Biol.* **263**: 551-567.

Schmiedl, A., Breitling, F., Winter, C.H., Queitsch, I., and Dübel, S., 2000, Effects of unpaired cysteines on yield, solubility and activity of different recombinant antibody constructs expressed in *E. coli. J. Immunol. Methods* **242**: 101-114.

Schwenk, J.M., Stoll, D., Templin, M.F., and Joos, T.O., 2002, Cell microarrays: an emerging technology for the characterization of antibodies. *Biotechniques*, **Suppl**, 54-61.

Sheets, M. D., Amersdorfer, P., Finnern, R., Sargent, P., Lindqvist, E., Schier, R., Hemingsen, G., Wong, C., Gerhardt, J. C. and Marks, J. D., 1998, Efficient construction of a large nonimmune phage antibody library: the production of high-affinity human single-chain antibodies to protein antigens. *Proc. Natl. Acad. Sci. USA* **95**: 6157 – 6162.

Siegel, R.W., Allen, B., Pavlik, P., Marks, J. D. and Bradbury, A., 2000, Mass spectral analysis of a protein complex using single-chain antibodies selected on a peptide target: applications to functional genomics. *J. Mol. Biol.* **302**:285-293.

Simmons, L.C. and Yansura, D.G., 1996, Translational level is a critical factor for the secretion of heterologous proteins in *Escherichia coli*. *Nat. Biotechnol.* **14**: 629-634.

Simmons, L.C., Reilly, D., Klimowski, L., Raju, T.S., Meng, G., Sims, P., Hong, K., Shields, R.L., Damico, L.A., Rancatore, P. and Yansura, D.G., 2002, Expression of full-length immunoglobulins in *Escherichia coli*: rapid and efficient production of aglycosylated antibodies. *J. Immunol. Methods* **263**: 133-147.

Skerra, A. and Plückthun, A., 1988, Assembly of a functional immunoglobulin Fv fragment in *Escherichia coli*. *Science* **240**: 1038-1041.

Smith, C.W., Marlin, S.D., Rothlein, R., Toman, C. and Anderson, D.C., 1989, Cooperative interactions of LFA-1 and Mac-1 with intercellular adhesion molecule-1 in facilitating adherence and transendothelial migration of human neutrophils *in vitro*. *J. Clin. Invest.* **83**: 2008-2017.

Söderlind, E., Strandberg, L., Jirholt, P., Kobayashi, N., Alexeiva, V., Aberg, A.-M., Nilsson, A., Jansson, B., Ohlin, M., Wingren, C., Danielson, L., Carlsson, R. and Borrebaeck, C.A.K., 2000, Recombining germline-derived CDR sequences for creating diverse single-framework antibody libraries. *Nat. Biotech.* **18**: 852 – 856.

Spirin, A.S., Baranov, V.I., Ryabova, L.A., Ovodov, S.Y. and Alakhov, Y.B., 1988, A continuous cell-free translation system capable of producing polypeptides in high yield. *Science* **242**: 1162-1164.

Sun, C., Kilburn, D., Lukashin, A., Crowell, T., Gardner, H., Brundiers, R., Diefenbach, B. and Carulli, J.P., 2003, Kirrel2, a novel immunoglobulin superfamily gene expressed primarily in beta cells of the pancreatic islets. *Genomics* **82**: 130-142.

Sun, J., Pons, J., and Craik, C.S., 2003, Potent and selective inhibition of membrane-type serine protease 1 by human single-chain antibodies. *Biochemistry* **42**: 892-900.

Sykes, K.F. and Johnston, S.A., 1999, Linear expression elements: a rapid, *in vivo*, method to screen for gene functions. *Nat. Biotechnol.* **17**: 355-359.

Takeuchi, T., Harris, J.L., Huang, W., Yan, K.W., Coughlin, S.R. and Craik, C.S., 2000, Cellular localization of membrane-type serine protease 1 and identification of protease-activated receptor-2 and single-chain urokinase-type plasminogen activator as substrates. *J. Biol. Chem.* **275**: 26333-26342.

Templin, M.F., Stoll, D., Schrenk, M., Traub, P.C., Vohringer, C.F. and Joos, T.O., 2002, Protein microarray technology. *Trends Biotechnol.* **20**: 160-166.

Tey, B.T., Singh, R.P., Piredda, L., Piacentini, M. and Al Rubeai, M., 2000, Bcl-2 mediated suppression of apoptosis in myeloma NS0 cultures. *J. Biotechnol.* **79**, 147-159.

Truman, J.-P., Ericson, M.L., Choqueux-Seebold, J.M., Charron, D.J. and Mooney, N.A., 1994, Lymphocyte programmed cell death is mediated via HLA class II DR. *Intl. Immunol.* **6**: 887-896.

Vaickus, L., Jones, V.E., Morton, C.L., Whitford, K. and Bacon, R.N., 1989, Antiproliferative mechanism of anti-class II monoclonal antibodies. *Cell Immunol.* **119**: 445-458.

Van Seventer, G.A., Shimizu, Y., Horgan, K.J. and Shaw, S., 1990, The LFA-1 ligand ICAM-1 provides an important costimulatory signal for T cell receptor-mediated activation of resting T cells. *J. Immunol.* **144**: 4579-4586.

Vaughan , T. J., Williams, A. J., Pritchard, K., Osbourn, J. K., Pope, A. R., Earnshaw, J. C., McCafferty, J., Hodits, R. A., Wilton, J. and Johnson K. S., 1996, Human antibodies with sub-nanomolar affinities isolated from a large non-immunized phage display library. *Nature Biotech.* **14**: 309 – 314.

Venter, J. C. and Adams, M. D., 1993. WO 93/00353.

Venturi, M., Seifert, C. and Hunte, C., 2002, High level production of functional antibody Fab fragments in an oxidizing bacterial cytoplasm. *J. Mol. Biol.* **315**: 1-8.

Vidovic, D., Falcioni, F., Siklodi, B., Belunis, C.J., Bolin, D.R., Ito, K. and Nagy Z.A., 1995, Down-regulation of class II major histocompatibility complex molecules on antigen presenting cells by antibody fragments. *Eur. J. Immunol.* **25**: 3349-3355.

Vidovic, D. and Toral, J., 1998, Selective apoptosis of neoplastic cells by the HLA-DR-specific monoclonal antibody. *Cancer Lett.* **128**: 127-135.

Virnekäs, B., Ge, L., Plückthun, A., Schneider, K.C., Wellnhofer, G. and Moroney, S.E., 1994, Trinucleotide phosphoramidites: ideal reagents for the synthesis of mixed oligonucleotides for random mutagenesis. *Nucl. Acids Res.* **22**: 5600-5607.

Voutsadakis, I.A., 2002, Gemtuzumab Ozogamicin (CMA-676, Mylotarg) for the treatment of CD33+ acute myeloid leukemia. *Anticancer Drugs* **13**: 685-692.

Waldmann, T.A., Levy, R. and Coller, B.S., 2000, Emerging therapies: spectrum of applications of monoclonal antibody therapy. *Hematology (Am. Soc. Hematol. Educ. Program),* 394-408.

Wall, J.G. and Plückthun, A., 1999, The hierarchy of mutations influencing the folding of antibody domains in *Escherichia coli. Protein Eng.* **12**: 605-611.

Walter, G., Bussow, K., Lueking, A. and Glokler, J., 2002, High-throughput protein arrays: prospects for molecular diagnostics. *Trends Mol. Med.* **8**: 250-253.

Watters, J.M., Telleman, P. and Junghans, R.P., 1997, An optimised method for cell-based phage display panning. *Immunotechnology* **3**: 21-29.

Webster, M.K. and Donoghue, D.J., 1997, Enhanced signaling and morphological transformation by a membrane-localized derivative of the fibroblast growth factor receptor 3 kinase domain. *Trends Genet.* **13**: 178-182.

Weir, A.N. and Bailey, N.A., 1997, Process for obtaining antibodies utilizing heat treatment. US 5,665,866.

Weir, A.N., Nesbitt, A., Chapman, A.P., Popplewell, A.G., Antoniw, P. and Lawson, A.D., 2002, Formatting antibody fragments to mediate specific therapeutic functions. *Biochem. Soc. Trans.* **30**: 512-516.

Willuda, J., Honegger, A., Waibel, R., Schubiger, P.A., Stahel, R., Zangemeister-Wittke, U. and Plückthun, A., 1999, High thermal stability is essential for tumour targeting of antibody fragments: engineering of a humanized anti-epithelial glycoprotein-2 (epithelial cell adhesion molecule) single-chain Fv fragment. *Cancer Res.* **59**: 5758-5767.

Willuda, J., Kubetzko, S., Waibel, R., Schubiger, P.A., Zangemeister-Wittke, U. and Plückthun, A., 2001, Tumour targeting of mono-, di-, and tetravalent anti-p185(HER-2) miniantibodies multimerised by self-associating peptides. *J. Biol. Chem.* **276**: 14385-14392.

Wörn, A. and Plückthun, A., 1999, Different equilibrium stability behaviour of scFv fragments: identification, classification, and improvement by protein engineering. *Biochemistry* **38**: 8739-8750.

Wörn, A. and Plückthun, A., 2001, Stability engineering of antibody single-chain Fv fragments. *J. Mol. Biol.* **305**: 989-1010.

Yang, W., Green, K., Pinz-Sweeney, S., Briones, A.T., Burton, D.R. and Barbas III, C.F., 1995, CDR walking mutagenesis for the affinity maturation of a potent human anti-HIV-1 antibody into the picomolar range. *J. Mol. Biol.* **254**: 392-403.

Chapter 3

ACHIEVING APPROPRIATE GLYCOSYLATION DURING THE SCALEUP OF ANTIBODY PRODUCTION

X. K. Deng[1], T. Shantha Raju[2] and K. John Morrow, Jr[1].
[1]*Meridian Bioscience, 3471 River Hills Drive, Cincinnati, OH 45244, USA and* [2]*CarboWorld, 1010 Haddon Drive, San Mateo, CA 94402, USA*

1. INTRODUCTION

Glycosylation is the most extensive and variable of mammalian post-translational modifications with profound implications for folding, stability, pharmacokinetics, antigenicity and biological activity of proteins. In the last several decades, improvements in the technology for analyzing protein glycosylation and measuring its biological effects have revolutionized the discipline of "glycobiology". Thus, extremely subtle alterations in glycoproteins can now be detected, and appropriate modifications brought about which were nearly impossible 20 years ago.

The technology of glycosylation is most relevant to investigators who intend to use antibodies *in vivo*, either in humans or in animal protocols. Antibody molecules belong to the immunoglobulin family, a majority of which are glycoproteins. Therefore, for those who need to perform procedures requiring the binding of mAbs to target proteins or Fc-receptors, absolute fidelity in the reconstruction of glycosylation pattern is essential. With the number of antibodies in clinical use steadily increasing, the biological significance of antibody glycosylation has gained importance for the biotechnology industry. Furthermore, the growing demand for antibody therapeutics is driving the need to expand capacity, with its attendant risks to fidelity of glycosylation, as the industry moves products from the level of research production to large scale (grams to kilograms) capacity, and eventually hundreds of kilograms.

2.   GLYCOSYLATION OF IMMUNOGLOBULIN MOLECULES AND ITS EFFECT ON ANTIBODY FUNCTION

2.1   Technology for the detection of glycosylation

The technology for complex carbohydrate analysis has been reviewed by Jenkins and Curling (1994), who stress that dramatic technical improvements now make continuous monitoring of glycosylation changes a reality. Rapid and highly sensitive analytical methods allow glycan structures to be determined in 1 or 2 days, and offer the possibility of monitoring carbohydrate changes in real time during fermentation. Mass spectrometry has made definitive structural analysis feasible within days of sampling, with obvious implications for regulatory authorities concerned with glycoprotein batch consistency.

2.1.1   Electrophoretic separations

Basic information concerning the presence or the absence of glycans has traditionally been obtained through electrophoretic techniques such as SDS-PAGE. This approach exploits a combination of commercially available polyacrylamide gels, endo- and exoglycosidase treatment, and "western" or dot blots employing specific lectins as detection agents. However, care must be taken to perform the analysis on highly glycosylated protein to avoid confounding the procedure with substantial smearing of electrophoretic bands.

Poor resolution is particularly a problem when analyzing products secreted into serum-based media or from intracellular components recovered from cell lysates. Gel analysis detects variable N-glycosylation and often site occupancy, but has limited value for detecting microheterogeneity of oligosacchride chains. Also, the negative charges due to sialic acid residues on many glycan structures may result in inaccurate mass assignments deduced from migration on SDS-PAGE gels. Similar shortcomings apply to isoelectric focusing for addressing gross heterogeneity in different batches of product (Jenkins and Curling, 1994).

Capillary electrophoresis (Koyama, et al, 2003) is an alternative new technology with its use of narrow bore capillaries to perform separations and high voltage to generate electro-osmotic and electrophoretic flow of buffer solutions and ionic species. It can be adapted to run in various modes (e.g. zone electrophoresis, isoelectric focusing, isotachophoresis, or micellar electrokinetic chromatography), providing a wide spectrum of analytical capabilities for resolving glycoproteins and glycopeptides. Capillary electrophoresis requires only small amount of samples, and glycoforms can be quantified by integrating the peaks detected by the UV or fluorescence detection.

Fluorophore-assisted carbohydrate electrophoresis (Robbe, et al, 2003) is an alternative approach to analyse glycoproteins, in which the total glycan moiety is released in a single step. The generated oligosaccharides are derivatized either with a hydrophobic fluorophore, and the resulting fluorescent derivatives separated by high-resolution gel electrophoresis. AMAC derivatization allows a separation of neutral and charged oligosaccharides without prior fractionation. Analysis of the products by mass spectrometry allows the rapid structural characterization of each glycan in terms of monosaccharide composition and sequence. This technique is accurate for screening heterogeneous glycan mixtures down to the picomolar range.

2.1.2   Chromatography

More precise structural analysis requires the cleavage of the glycoprotein molecule into smaller components, through proteolytic digestion and chromatographic resolution to generate glycopeptides, or to chemically degrade the peptide backbone. Analytic approaches achieved by generating glycopeptides are becoming increasingly important as more products are shown to exhibit clear differences between individual glycosylation sites on the same protein. However, glycosylation profiles may influence the efficiency of proteolytic digestion, leading to distortions in quantifying the relative amount of glycoforms within each glycoprotein.

Glycopeptides are commonly resolved from other peptides using reverse-phase high performance liquid chromatography (Rabina, et al, 2001). The oligosaccharides can then be removed from the peptide using the enzyme peptide N-glycosidase F (PNGaseF). This enzyme cleaves most common mammalian N-linked oligosaccharides. Additionally, hydrazinolysis has become an alternative method for releasing both N- and O-linked glycans, whose profiles could be obtained by high pH anion exchange chromatography with pulsed amperometric detection (HPAEC-PAD) or by other chromatographic and electrophoretic methods. Neutral monosaccharides, amino sugars, and charged sugars can be analyzed using HPAEC-PAD with sensitivity in the picomolar range. These techniques along with exoglycosidase digestion and mass spectral characterization confirm the structures of various oligosaccharides.

High performance liquid chromatography combined with electrospray ionization mass spectrometry is an elegant tool for resolving oligosaccharides of great complexity. Wang, et al. (2003) analysed a murine IgM by this method, determining that 5 N-glycosylation sites possessed a wealth of diverse glycosylation patterns, up to 20 residues in some cases, including complex and hybrid type oligosaccharides.

2.1.3   Nuclear magnetic resonance (NMR)

NMR technology, widely applied today in structural analysis (Rudisser and Jahnke, 2002), allows the determination of unambiguous structures of oligosaccharides derived from glycoproteins. A one dimensional ^{1}H-NMR spectrum can be used as a fingerprint to identify a specific glycan structure by comparing it to a database of NMR spectra. This widely used method requires only about 50 nmol of material, while more sophisticated forms of NMR, using multi dimension and dipolar corrections, used to determine specific linkages between saccharide units, require considerably more sample.

2.1.4   Mass spectrometry

Fast atom bombardment mass spectrometry (FAB-MS), used to deduce glycan structures of a number of glycoproteins (Silverman, et al, 2003), requires a relatively large amount of pure sample. Its exceptional mass accuracy can be used to obtain semi-quantitative data on the degree of glycan occupancy at specific glycosylation sites within a particular glycoprotein. This is possible because glycan-substituted Asn residues are converted to Asp residues when cleaved by PNGaseF, resulting in a mass increase of 1Da compared to an unoccupied site. This type of analysis allows monitoring of the glycan occupancy status of individual N-glycosylation sites.

Alternatives to FAB-MS include electrospray ionization mass spectrometry (ES-MS) and/or matrix assisted laser desorption ionization time-of-flight mass spectrometry (MALDI-TOF-MS) techniques. The mass accuracy of this techniques is between 0.05-0.1%. ES-MS has the added advantage that it can be coupled directly to either CE or HPLC separation of glycoforms and released oligosaccharides. MALDI-TOF-MS instruments have become affordable to many more laboratories than FAB-MS. No derivatization of sample is required to obtain good glycan structural data on small amounts of protein. Even in the presence of small amounts of salts derived from buffer solutions there is no interfere with the procedure.

2.2　Types of glycosylated structures occurring in proteins

The effect of antibody glycosylation on biological function is pivotal for the biotechnology industry, as ~70% of subjects undergoing clinical development for therapeutic applications are antibodies (Jefferis and Lund, 1997). Oligosaccharides are essential for activation of effector functions leading to the destruction of pathogens. While the biological activity of some therapeutic glycoproteins (other than immunoglobulins) may not be dependent on glycosylation, the stability, pharmacokinetics, and antigenicity are altered by removal of the carbohydrate residues, with obvious implications for the pharmacological functions of these molecules.

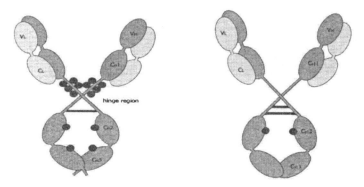

IgA1　　　　　　　　　IgG1

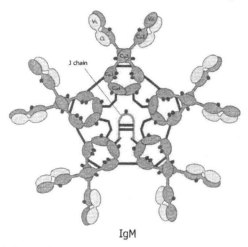

IgM

Figure 3.1. Glycosylation of the constant regions of the IgA, IgG and IgM molecules (small, dark spheres) From Das and Morrow (2002).

2.2.1   Glycosylation of the constant region of the antibody molecule

Antibodies contain 3-12% carbohydrates at conserved N-glycosylation sites located in the constant region of the heavy chains (Leibiger, et al., 1999). The Fc glycosylation site, a constant feature for all mammalian IgGs, occurs at a homologous position in human IgM, IgD and IgE molecules but not in IgA. Human IgM, IgA, IgE and IgD molecules bear additional N-linked oligosaccharide moieties attached to the constant domains of the heavy chains. IgD and IgA proteins also bear multiple O-linked sugars in their extended hinge regions, attached to hydroxyl groups of serine and/or threonine residues (see Figure 3.1). It has been estimated that ~30% of IgG molecules also contain N-glycosylation in the Fab region.

The Fc region of IgG molecule contains N-linked oligosaccharides at Asn297 on the β-4 bend of the inner (Fx) C_H2 domain face. This complex biantenary structure has a pentasaccharide 'core' (Man3GlcNAc2) and variable sugar residues, such as fucose, bisecting N-acetylglucosamine, galactose and sialic acid residues (Figure 3.2). This variability imparts a large repertoire of possibilities; moreover, glycosylation can be asymmetric allowing different oligosaccharide chains attached at each of the Asn297 residues. This results in a cornucopia of glycoforms; a total of (36*36)/2=648 structurally unique IgG molecules can occur.

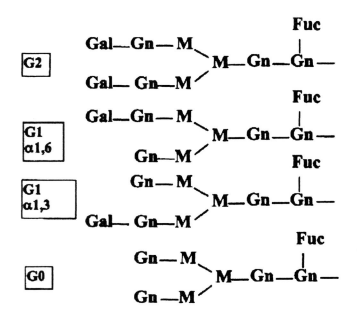

Figure 3.2. Varieties of glycosylation patterns.

While the heavy chain synthesized within a single antibody-secreting cell will not vary in its amino acid sequence (except with the C-terminal Lys content), glycosylation can result in the production of many different molecules within a single cell. The total number of combination was divided by two because of the two-fold symmetry of the molecule. All oligosaccharide species are encountered, with the exception of disialylated oligosaccharides, which may be absent or present at a very low level. The presence of additional glycosylation sites within the heavy chains of the other Ig isotypes means that the possible number of glycoforms is greatly expanded [Umana, et al., 1999; Lifely, et al., 1995].

2.2.2   Glycosylation within the variable region

IgG antibodies are usually not glycosylated in their variable regions (Leibiger, et al., 1999). However, in cases in which glycosylation does occur, low affinity antibodies might be enhanced in their binding by carbohydrate-induced conformational changes. Glycosylation in Fab regions is due to the presence of potential N-glycosylation sequence within either the V_L or V_H domains. DNA sequences of 83 human germline V_H gene segments produced five sequences that encoded potential N-glycosylation sites. However, none of these sequons were observed in 37 V_H protein sequences that were subjected to detailed analysis. The question of whether the germline gene from which these proteins were derived did encode a glycosylation sequon was not investigated. Fifteen of the 37 protein sequences did show potential glycosylation sequons which, it would appear, have resulted from somatic mutation and antigen selection [Jefferis and Lund, 1997].

Oligosaccharides in the variable region can affect antibody performance, as shown by a monoclonal murine anti-dextran antibody with a single oligosaccharide attachment site at residues 54, 58 or 60 in complementarity-determining region 2 (CDR2) which possessed dissimilar antigen-binding activities [Monica, et al, 1995]. The IgG glycans present in the F_c are (Dwek et al.,1995) mainly three types of complex biantennary oligosaccharides containing zero, one, or two galactose residues on their outer arms, commonly known as G0, G1, and G2, respectively (Figure 3.2). Within each class, there are four species that result from the presence or absence of core fucose and/or "bisecting" GlcNAc residues. Further heterogeneity arises as a result of sialylation of some terminal galactose residues. IgG's contains an average of 2.4 glycans (Youings et al., 1996), of which 2 are conserved at Asn 297 in the CH2 domain of the Fc region. These site-specific glycosylations demonstrate their complex role and the many levels at which immunoregulation can occur.

The additional oligosaccharides are located in the hypervariable regions in the Fab. The glycosylation of IgG Fc is important both in its normal physiological role and in certain disease pathologies (Wormald, et al, 1997).

2.2.3   Physico-chemical effect of antibody glycosylation

Biophysical studies have suggested that the Fc oligosaccharides have the same dynamic properties as the C_{H2} domains. In contrast, X-ray crystallographic studies of mouse IgG Fab show only poorly defined electron density at the N-glycosylation site (Stanfield et al., 1990), indicating oligosaccharide mobility or disorder within the crystal structure. Electron spin resonance spin labeling studies on IgM Fab and intact IgM (Lapuk et al., 1984) have shown the *N*-glycans to have a much higher degree of mobility than the peptide. Structural investigation of the differences between IgG glycoforms has so far been limited to circular dichroism studies of normal and rheumatoid IgG. Differences between the circular dichroism spectra of intact normal and rheumatoid IgG have been interpreted in terms of a structural anomaly in the hinge region of rheumatoid IgG (Johnson et al., 1974), while circular dichroism studies on immune complexes from rheumatoid patients have suggested that only a portion of rheumatoid IgG contains these unusual structural determinants (Uesson & Hansson, 1982).

2.3   Enzymatic reactions responsible for glycosylation

Addition of glycosyl residues to protein is brought about by co-translation of preformed mannose, glucose, and *N*-acetylglucosamine from a dolichol intermediate to the growing polypeptide chain. The terminal glucoses are bound by the chaperone calnexin and must be removed to allow transit through the endoplasmic reticulum (see Figure 3.3). Normal human serum IgG displays a cornucopia of diversity, yielding up to thirty different structures (Rudd et al, 1991) resulting from variation in core substitution of fucose and/or bisecting *N*-acetylglucosamine (GlcNAc) and in processing of the outer arms of the biantennary sugar. Mouse cells can add an additional terminal galactose with a novel alpha 1,3 linkage. This residue might be immunogenic in humans and over 1% of serum IgG is directed against the Gal alpha 1,3-Gal beta 1,4-GlcNAc epitope, possibly as a consequence of its presence on enteric bacteria. Hamedah et al., (1996) demonstrated that an acellular Klebsiella pneumoniae sonicate could add ^{3}H-UDP-Gal to human RBCs.

CHO cells as well as human, ape, and Old World monkey cells lack the enzyme required to attach the alpha 1,3 galactosyl structure (Borrebaeck et al., 1993).

3. IMPLICATIONS OF GLYCOSYLATION FOR LARGE SCALE PRODUCTION OF ANTIBODY MOLECULES

Progress in understanding the effect of glycosylation was limited until recently largely due to the complexity of methods used for the analysis of oligosaccharides. Bernstein (1987) reviewed glycosylation of plasma proteins, and cited a wide range of assay methods available at that time, with affinity chromatography, isoelectric focusing, and spectrophotometric tools providing the best accuracy and versatility. Since then, improvements in technology make it possible to detect subtle changes occurring through different production methods and place greater burden on the biotechnology industry to produce glycoprotein therapeutics in a consistent manner during the course of upscaling to industrial volumes.

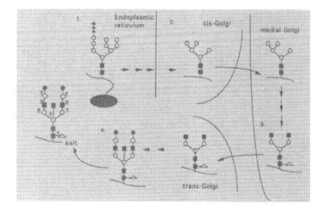

Figure 3.3. Processing pathway of oligosaccharides to a complex biantennary form (From Yoo, et al., 2002). Symbols: glucose (▲); mannose (O); *N*-acetylglucosamine (■); fucose (△); galactose (◊); sialic acid (■)

3.1 Glycosylation of antibodies generated in mouse ascites.

Glycosylation, a complex post-translational event, can be influenced by a variety of factors such as culture conditions, medium supplements and purification procedures. Thus, *in vitro* methods enable the desired glycosylation structure to be obtained by making an appropriate choice of these factors. For example, mAbs with a glycosylation pattern of the biantennary complex oligosaccharide type are often favored. While this goal can be easily achieved in hollow fibre bioreactors, antibodies produced by the ascites method cannot be influenced by their glycosylation pattern, which may vary from mouse to mouse.

Production of ascites in mice for therapeutic purposes is not appropriate as it does not provide the necessary fidelity of glycosylation patterns for introduction into patients. Nonetheless, for non-therapeutic applications, ascites preparations are still in wide use. The *in vivo* procedures entail the use of mice or rats (Marx, 1998), injected with hybridoma cells, which then multiply in the peritoneal cavity, forming ascitic fluid, a rich source of the secreted antibody. The main advantage of this strategy is the extremely high yield of antibody, approximately in the range of 1-20mg/ml. However, there are a number of disadvantages, including the ethical issues involved in developing ascites tumors and the reduced immunoreactivity of antibodies (around 60-70%) due to contamination with cytokines and other circulating proteins.

3.2   Glycosylation of antibodies produced by *in vitro* cell culture methods

Hormones, culture method, age of the culture, pH, buffers and serum components can all affect glycosylation patterns. Biosynthesis of oligosaccharides is a multistep process and numerous enzymes are involved, including glycosyltransferases and glycosidases (Hiatt, 1992). These enzymes are often competing with each other for a single substrate, with the result that the products are a microheterogeneous array of glycoproteins with frequently truncated terminal Gal and GlcNAc residues along with sialic acid (Sia) residues.

3.2.1   Mammalian cell culture parameters affecting glycosylation

There are differences in glycosylation between human and rodent cells. Bisecting GlcNAc residues are present in ~10-20% of human IgGs but CHO cells lack the GnT-III enzyme required for its addition. Another striking difference between human and rodent cells is the form of sialic acid utilized; 25% of oligosaccharides of human IgG have terminal N-acetylneuraminic acid while N-glycolyneuraminic acid occurs in mice. Chimeric mouse/human IgG3 may contain both (Borys, et al., 1994).

Culture conditions may produce IgGs that are glycosylated at positions different from those obtained in mouse ascites fluid. For example, an IgG has been found to contain unusual mannose moieties at all glycosylation sites under certain culture conditions. This antibody has an increased clearance rate *in vivo* because of its binding to the mannose receptors in the liver. Many mammalian cell lines have been used to express recombinant proteins because they have the ability to carry out normal post-translational modifications.   Myeloma expression systems producing genetically engineered Abs have been used successfully for a variety of diagnostic, imaging and therapeutic applications.

Myeloma cell lines are easy to grow in suspension culture and are adaptable for large-scale production (Yoo et al, 2002). The availability of a variety of commercial serum-free media for production of therapeutic Mabs is another major advantage of this system. The most commonly used cell lines are P3X63Ag8.653, Sp2/0-Ag14 and NSO/1, all of which derived from the mineral oil-induced plasmacytomas developed many years ago by Potter at NIH (Potter and Lieberman, 1970). Most IgG molecules produced by normal human B lymphocytes possess a bisecting GlcNAc residue β1-4 linked to the central β-linked mannose of the Man3 core structure. Bisecting GlcNAc has been shown to enhance the ability of IgG to mediate antigen dependent cellular cytotoxicity. But these bisecting GlcNAc moieties are rarely seen in IgG's produced in myeloma cells.   There are other heterogeneities between human glycan and mouse glycan, most of them occurring in terminal residues. For example N-glycolylneuramic acid (NeuGc), a derivative of N-acetylneuraminic acid (NeuAc), is an oncofetal antigen. Antibodies from mouse or human–mouse hybridomas contain more NeuGc than NeuAc (Monica, et al, 1995), although it is not usually encountered in adult humans.

Glycosylation in these cell lines always follow that pattern characteristic of the mouse, rather than the human parental line (Monica et al., 1995). They lack bisecting N-acetylglucosamine, and exhibit lower sialylation and galactosylation, some are oligomannose type or monoantennary complex-type and some contain N-glycolylneuraminic acid and additional α galactose residues not present in human IgG (Lund et al, 1993: Jefferis et al., 1992). Different cell lines may add different terminal sugar residues to the antibody molecule. For example hybridomas and mouse–human heterohybridomas synthesize glycans terminating in Gal alpha 1,3–Gal beta 1,4–GlcNAc (Borrebaeck, 1993). But other rodent lines such as mouse NSO or rat Y3 myelomas producing humanized Abs do not add Gal alpha 1,3-Gal beta 1,4-GlcNAc (Lifely et al., 1995). CHO cells perform glycosylation steps in a fashion comparable to human cells, and are therefore favored for production of therapeutic proteins.

The glycosylation profiles from antibodies produced in NS0 cells are very similar to that from CHO. However further analysis after exoglycosidase treatment suggested underglycosylation. The difference in glycosylation of the various antibody preparations did not affect their ability to bind to the CD52 antigen. Antibodies produced by the YO cell line showed increased ADCC activity compared to CHO antibodies, possibly due to the presence of bisecting GlcNAc in the YO antibody. By contrast, no difference was found between the antibodies in their performance in the monocyte killing assay.

These results suggest that major differences in antibody glycosylation occur between cell lines and growth under different culture conditions.

But program designers may find themselves in a "Catch 22" situation, since when the culture conditions are optimized to maximize yield, the CHO cells often encounter difficulties with the whole glycosylation process and generate truncated oligosaccharide chains instead of branched chains with several sugar moieties. Manipulations such as addition of butyrate cause an increase in cell growth rate but can lead to the induction of certain glycosyltransferases thereby altering the sequence of the carbohydrate structures (Nakao, et al. 1990). The addition of butyrate induced the activity of core-2-GlcNActransferase of the O-glycosylation pathway therefore reduced the amount of α 2, 6-sialic acid (Shah et al., 1992).

Further, CHO cells are known to lack the functional enzyme α 2, 6-sialytransferase, leading to exclusively α 2,3 terminal sialic acid residues (Lee et al., 1989). Most mouse cell lines possess both functional α 2,3- and α 2,6- sialytransferases, a property they share with human cells. But they also express the alpha 1,3- galactosyltransferase which might be immunogenic to humans.

Finally, expression in a human cell line does not guarantee a reproducible glycosylation profile. This is because glycosylation changes with the culture conditions and also with the cell age.

3.2.2   Effect of varying culture conditions

Different culture conditions also influence the structure of the N-linked oligosaccharides. Most comparisons of the glycosylation profiles resulting from different methods of cell culture have been made on hybridoma-produced immunoglobulins. A monoclonal IgG$_1$ was produced by the murine hybridoma 3.8.6 as ascites, in serum free medium and in serum supplemented medium (Patel et al 1992). The ascites-derived material contained no sialic acid residues while the serum-free material contained the highest sialic acid content. Antibodies derived from serum containing media had an intermediate sialic acid content and a lower amount of outer arm galactosylation than the other two preparations.

Kumpel et al (1994) described the glycosylation of human IgG monoclonal anti-D (the Rh factor responsible for newborn hemolytic anemia) produced by EBV-transformed B-lymphoblastoid cells. The Mab was produced in serum free medium in low density static culture and also at high density in a hollow fiber bioreactor. The low density Mab contained >70% digalactosylated structures. The high density Mab, by contrast, contained relatively high levels (over 50%) of monogalactosyl oligosaccharides. The low density-generated Mab was more active than the high density form in monocyte and K cell mediated lysis of erythrocytes in antigen dependent cell cytotoxicity assays. This is due to the difference in level of terminal galactoses between Mabs produced under the two different sets of conditions. These results suggest that the low and high-density culture conditions affect the glycosylation of antibodies, possibly due to the presence of cytokines in the high density medium.

In support of this contention, addition of IL6 to the medium reduced the N-acetylglucosaminyltransferase-III (GnT-III) activity in myeloma cell cultures but increased GnT-IV and GnT-V activity, leading to altered glycosylation profiles. It has been observed that during the process of cell adaption from suspension to serum free medium, endogenous fucosyltransferase could be activated resulting in the expression of the oncofetal antigen, sialylated Lewis-x. The sialylation differences occurred between low and high density Mab. The overall outcome was that the high density glycosylation profiles and functional activity were more similar to normal serum IgG.

It was also shown that antibodies produced by hybridomas grown in serum containing medium generated a higher proportions of terminal galactose residues than those grown in protein free medium. Further, the different culture conditions used in this study resulted in less significant effects on CHO antibody glycosylation compared with the other two cell lines.

Glucose concentrations have been found to affect the degree of glycosylation of Mabs produced by human hybridomas in batch culture. Such changes may be due to limiting glucose. In a study of glucose concentrations in the medium. In the study of limited chemostat cultures, the cells grow at low rates and produce increased levels of nonglycosylated interferon (Hayter, et al, 1993). Addition of glucose leads to a rapid improvement in the proportion of fully glycosylated product and also increased the cell growth. Once the glucose injection was stopped, the glycosylation decreased as before. Therefore, cell culture conditions can influence both the extent and type of the carbohydrate on antibodies produced in myeloma cell lines (Jenkins et al, 1996).

Other factors affecting glycosylation include oxygen concentration (Kunkel, et al., 2000). Murine hybridoma cells were grown in serum free continuous culture at steady state dissolved oxygen concentrations of 10%, 50%, and 100% of air saturation in both LH series 210 (LH) and New Brunswick scientific (NBS) Celligen Bioreactors. The lower dissolved oxygen reduced the level of galactosylation. Higher level of sialylation of Mab glycans in the NBS bioreactor than in the LH bioreactors occurred at all three concentrations. These results indicates that normally identical steady state condition in different chemostat bioreactors may still lead to some differences in glycosylation, possibly due to the particular architectures of the bioreactors and the design of their respective monitoring and control systems.

Immunoglobulin types produced under different methods have also been investigated by Gauny et al (1991). These workers demonstrated that human monoclonal IgM produced by a human-human-mouse trioma in cell culture had a more rapid clearance rate than the same antibody made in mouse ascites. Monica et al (1993) compared the biochemical characterization of human IgG produced in both ascites and *in vitro* cell culture and found notable differences in the distribution of common structures in the two HPAE-PAD maps. Further, reverse phase peptide maps of tryptic digests of the ascites and cell culture IgM show significant differences.

Other physical parameters of cell culture affecting glycosylation profiles include pH levels outside the range of 6.9 to 8.2, which increases underglycosylation, and high ammonium ion which may affect the sialyltransferases activity present in the Golgi thus resulting in reduced sialic acids residues in G-CSF (Anderson, et al., 1994). Increased ammonium ion also reduced the extent of recombinant placental lactogen N-glycosylation by CHO cells, but this was dependent on the pH (Borys, 1994).

Schenerman et al (1999) carried out extensive biochemical and functional testing of a humanized monoclonal antibody (Synagis) to evaluate cell line stability, support process validation, and to demonstrate "comparability" during the course of process development. Results showed that there was a different pattern of glycosylation during the early stages of bioreactor culture. No other changes in microheterogeneity were apparent for the other culture conditions studied. Samples taken from the production bioreactor on days 5, 11 and 18 were based on a typical 18–22-day cell culture production process. As the harvest time impacted the final oligosaccharide profile, it was vital to maintain in-process controls and specifications to assure the consistency of product. It appears that upscaling can be controlled to retain comparable glycosylation, resulting in a predictable and reproducible monoclonal antibody product.

3.3   Bacteria

Bacteria lack much of the complex and variable glycosylation mechanisms of eukaryotes. Although N-linked protein glycosylation is the most abundant posttranslational modification of secretory proteins in eukaryotes, bacterial expression systems have limited capacity to glycosylate proteins as shown by recent studies in *E. coli* and other species. Wacker, et al (2002) found an N-linked glycosylation system in the bacterium *Campylobacter jejuni* and transferred it into *Escherichia coli*. The bacterial N-glycan differs structurally from its eukaryotic counterparts, but the authors suggest that it could function as a universal N-linked glycosylation cassette in *E. coli* for research and industrial applications.

E. coli contains its own endogenous glycosylation capability. A novel glycoprotein has been isolated and purified from the non-pathogenic strain of this organism (Kumar et al., 2003). This glycoprotein, Gp45, was isolated with sodium deoxycholate and further purified on DEAE-Sephadex A-25 to homogeneity. It contained 60% carbohydrate and 40% protein.

Although other bacterial strains such as *Neisseria meningitis* have recently been shown to O-glycosylate certain of their endogenous proteins, the trisaccharide added is different from the O-linked sugars found in eukaryotes (Jenkins, et al, 1996). Hamadeh, et al (1996) characterized alpha 1,3 galactosyltransferases (alpha 1,3 GT) from Klebsiella, finding at least four galactosyltransferases that can add an alpha Gal to human cell surface acceptor structures. These enzymes can form alpha 1,3 Gal structures on human red blood corpuscles that bind anti-Gal, creating "autoimmune" senescence-associated RBC epitopes and possibly contributing to senescence in humans.

3.4   Yeast

Jenkins et al (1996) have explored yeast systems for the production of glycosylated recombinant antibodies. The hypermannosylation (addition of a large number of mannose residues to the trimannosyl core oligosaccharide) is a common property of most yeast strains and can compromise the efficacy of recombinant proteins such as the hepatitis B vaccine. This can be prevented by expressing the polypeptide in mutant yeast strains such as mm-9 or the temperature-sensitive ngd-29 in which N- glycosylation is confined to core oligosaccharide residues with a limited mannose content (up to Man8GlcNAc). This strategy has been adopted for more effective vaccine production. There is also evidence to suggest that different O-glycosylation sites are used by yeast and mammalian cells.

3.5   Glycosylation in transgenic plants

Although tobacco is the traditional tool for foreign DNA introduction, many laboratories have perfected transfection techniques for common crop plants such as corn, soybean, alfalfa and rice (Hein et al., 1991). Hiatt et al (1992) reported the use of tobacco to synthesize antibodies that could protect against caries-causing bacteria when added to toothpaste.

Zeitlin et al (1998) have genetically engineered soybeans to produce a humanized monoclonal antibody for the development of a method of mucosal immunoprotection against sexually transmitted diseases. They compared a humanized anti-herpes simplex virus 2 (HSV-2) Mab expressed in mammalian cell culture with the same antibody expressed in soybeans. These Mabs were similar in their stability in human semen and cervical mucus over 24 h, their ability to diffuse in human cervical mucus, and their efficacy for prevention of vaginal HSV-2 infection in the mouse.

Hiatt (1992) reviewed the performance of antibodies expressed in plants, focusing on the IgG and alternative forms of immunoglobulin. In terms of lectin binding "plantibodies" act differently than the same antibodies generated in mouse ascites. Both heavy chain were bound by concanavalin A (specific for mannose and glucose binding). But the ascites-produced heavy chain was also recognized by *ricinus communis* (specific for terminal galactose) and wheat germ agglutinin (*N*-acetylglucosamine and terminal sialic acid). This finding indicates that plant glycans have different terminal sugar residues, an observation consistent with the absence of N-acetyl neuraminic acid in the plant systems.

Plant glycans were found to be resistant to endoglycosidase H, a property of complex carbohydrates processed in the Golgi apparatus. This finding indicates that the transgenic plant antibody is processed in a similar fashion to mammalian glycoprotein. In addition both glycans have approximately the same affinity for Con A since they were not distinguishable by competition with α-methyl mannoside. Das and Morrow (2002) summarized the work with plantibodies and other high quality engineered proteins in transgenic plants. Plant glycoproteins containing beta-linked xylose sugars may be immunogenic (see Figure 3.4), since they are recognized by IgE and could stimulate an allergenic response in humans. The issue is under study using a rodent model (Chargelegue et al., 2000). Mice were immunized subcutaneously with a recombinant mouse monoclonal antibody produced in tobacco, together with alum as adjuvant. Analyses by direct immunoassay, competition immunoassay and real-time surface plasmon resonance showed undetectable levels of antibody directed against both the protein and the glycan part of the plant recombinant antibody. These results have a relevance for the application of plant recombinant proteins as therapeutic agents and vaccines, but more extensive studies on human patients are required to resolve the issue.

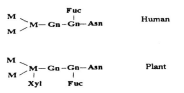

Figure 3.4. Major differences in glycosylation patterns between human and plant cells.

4. IMPLICATIONS OF ANTIBODY GLYCOSYLATION FOR THE BIOTECHNOLOGY INDUSTRY

4.1 Options for large-scale production of antibodies

For antibodies whose effector functions are dependent on the structure of their complex N-linked oligosaccharide, the potential of cell culture process variations to introduce structural heterogeneity to N-linked carbohydrates is a particular challenge for product consistency. There is still no specific FDA or cGMP document that deals with glycosylation of antibodies. At present most recombinant proteins intended for human therapy are accepted with some degree of glycosylation heterogeneity. But FDA officials have already pointed out it is important to develop appropriate analytical tests to ensure consistency between lots. This concern on the part of regulatory agencies indicates that the glycosylation status of products will need to be well established. The ability to manufacture an antibody with structurally consistent carbohydrates would be advantageous because it would allow maximal control over lot-to-lot analytical and biological variability.

In vitro methods enable the desired glycosylation structures to be obtained by making an appropriate choice of systems. Jenkins (1996) indicates that both the analytical techniques used to measure glycoprotein heterogeneity and methods used to control the biosynthetic pathways of glycosylation are being exhaustively investigated. Improvements in analytical procedures now offer the prospect of detailed glycan analysis during or soon after fermentation of recombinant cells. This together with a more detailed knowledge of the glycoprotein biosynthetic pathway, may lead to methods of controlling glycan heterogeneity using special media formulations or supplements during fermentation.

4.2 Use of recombinant technology for appropriate glycosylation

Cloning and analysis of glycosyltransferase genes is expediting the *in vitro* production of properly glycosylated proteins. These analyses highlight the differences between the glycosylation machinery of different cell types. Supplementing the cells' endogenous equipment with cloned glycosyltransferase genes has already been achieved for some enzymes, and this type of glycosylation engineering will complement the use of glycosylation mutants for the production of antibodies containing specific glycoforms. As the biological roles for specific glycan structures become apparent, it may be desirable to manipulate the host cells genetically or physiologically for the biased production of certain glycoforms.

Alternatively, downstream processing techniques may be developed to select for different glycoforms in the cell culture medium. Advances have been made to manipulate the culture conditions to obtain desired terminal sialylation of the product. The CHO cell line expresses a wide variety of recombinant proteins by transfection of the appropriate glycosyltransferases (Lee, et al., 1989). Substantial effort has been made to minimize the heterogeneity among different product lots (Stanley, 1992).

An antineuroblastoma chimeric IgG1, engineered in CHO cells with a tetracycline–regulated   expression   of   beta $(1,4)$–N–acetylglucosaminyltransferase III (GnTIII), catalyzed the formation of bisected GlcNAc containing oligosaccharides. This antibody conveyed antigen-dependent cell cytotoxicity, and this activity correlated with the level of constant region–associated, bisected GlcNAc containing complex oligosaccharides (Umana et al 1999). The new optimized Mabs exhibit substantial ADCC activity and, hence, may be useful for treatment of neuroblastoma. This strategy should be applicable to optimize the ADCC activity of other therapeutic IgGs.

Weikert et al (1999) engineered two CHO cell lines secreting different recombinant glycoproteins to express high levels of human beta 1,4-galactosyltransferase (GT) and/or alpha 2,3-sialyltransferase (ST). N-linked oligosaccharide structures synthesized by cells overexpressing the glycosyltransferases showed greater homogeneity compared with control cell lines. When GT was overexpressed, oligosaccharides terminating with GlcNAc were significantly reduced compared with controls, whereas overexpression of ST resulted in sialylation of ≥90% of available branches. As expected, GT overexpression resulted in reduction of oligosaccharides terminating with GlcNAc, whereas overexpression of ST resulted in sialylation of ≥90% of oligosaccharides. The more highly sialylated glycoproteins had a significantly longer mean residence time in a rabbit model.

This study showed an improvement in glycoprotein quality as a decrease in glycosylation heterogeneity resulting from an increase in the molar content of galactose and sialic acid. However, it is unclear at present what the "best" carbohydrate for each glycoprotein might be. An additional step in engineering recombinant glycoproteins may involve humanization of CHO oligosaccharides by coexpression of ST and/or the GlcNAc transferase-III enzyme, which is responsible for the addition of bisecting GlcNAc residue on oligosaccharides derived from humans and other species. Other investigators have attempted to overexpress ST in CHO and baby hamster kidney lines in an effort to produce more human type oligosaccharide structures. This enzyme has been shown to compete with the endogenous ST for the donor sugar cytidine monophosphate (CMP)-sialic acid (Jenkins, 1992).

It is currently unknown whether the presence of alpha 2, 6- as well as alpha 2, 3-linked sialic acids have any significance in terms of the biological or pharmacokinetic properties of glycoproteins. However, overexpression of glycosyltransferases can impact the quality of oligosaccharides on recombinant glycoproteins and hence suggest that it is possible to use host cells with specifically tailored glycosynthetic profiles to predetermine the composition of the N-linked oligosaccharides produced during large-scale mammalian cell culture.

Proteins with insufficient sialic acid are subject to drastically reduced half-life in circulation. By sialylating these molecules using *in vitro* glycosylation methods it is possible to produce a properly sialylated product. The reduction in half-life is the result of terminal galactose residues on the oligosaccharide structure, which allows binding to the asialoglycoprotein receptor that is present in the liver. The capping of the terminal galactose group with sialic acid prevents binding to asialoglycoprotein and subsequent clearance from the circulation in the liver.

As mentioned above, glycosyltransferases are useful reagents for *in vitro* synthesis of oligosaccharides and glycoconjugates. Raju et al. (2001) used a combination of beta 1,4 GT and alpha 2,3 ST to regalactosylate and resialylate glycoprotein glycans containing terminal GlcNAc and Gal in a single reaction step, to reduce microheterogeneity and to increase the level of terminal sialylation. Results of the combination reaction were comparable to the results of stepwise regalactosylation and resialylation reactions obtained in two separate steps. The in vitro glycosylation of therapeutic glycoproteins using multiple enzymes in a single reaction is useful and efficient in producing homogeneously glycosylated therapeutic glycoproteins. This type of in vitro glycosylation reactions can be very easily scaled up for industrial production of therapeutic glycoproteins.

5.   FUTURE OUTLOOK

5.1   Transgenic animals

There are relatively few studies on the glycosylation of recombinant proteins expressed in the milk of transgenic animals. Choi et al (2001) investigated bovine beta-casein expressed in transgenic mouse milk. The purified beta-casein showed an N-linked oligosaccharide attached to Asn68 and different lectin binding profiles compared with the same protein expressed in yeast. The mouse-expressed beta-casein oligosaccharide structure is different in the mammary gland of mouse than the reported glycosylated beta-casein expressed in *Pichia pastoris*.

The published data on glycoproteins produced in transgenic goats indicate a similar but significantly different glycosylation pattern than human and CHO cells. Interferon-γ expressed in transgenic mice showed a greater proportion of truncated and oligomannose structures at the Asn97 site compared to IFN-γ expressed in CHO cells, although the level of glycosylation site occupancy was increased. Glycoprotein can be remodeled in situ by the transgenic expression of additional glycosyltransferases in the mouse mammary gland. Among many systems used for recombinant protein production under investigation, the milk of transgenic cattle has been proposed as an attractive vehicle for large-scale production (van Berkel, et al, 2002). Recombinant human lactoferrin (rhLF), an iron-binding glycoprotein involved in innate host defense, has been produced in bovine milk at gram/L levels. Although natural hLF and rhLF underwent differential N-linked glycosylation, they displayed equivalent behavior in different in vivo infection models employing immunocompetent and leukocytopenic mice, and showed similar localization at sites of infection. Thus, transgenic cattle may be used effectively for the large-scale production of biopharmaceuticals.

5.2   Very large scale production

It is conceivable that some applications might call for very large amounts of antibodies, perhaps in the range of hundreds or even thousands of kilograms. These may include wide spread use of therapeutic antibodies for cancer or other chronic applications, including autoimmune conditions. Other megascale applications could include the use of antibodies for industrial applications, including catalytic antibodies, and topical applications, such as toothpaste containing antibodies directed against periodontic or caries-causing bacteria (Abiko, 2000).

5.2.1   Options for large scale antibody production

With increasing demands for very large amounts of perfectly glycosylated therapeutic antibodies, biotech companies are moving to greater and greater capacities. Although it is currently the method of choice, mammalian cell culture has a number of inherent limitations. These include limitation of scale, up to approximately 50,000 liters, long culture periods, and limits in availability of medium components. These factors can limit the production to a level of perhaps 500 kg per year of antibody. In addition, the capital costs are high, and the potential for contamination with adventious agents exists.

Bacterial antibody production facilities on the other hand can generate multi-ton yields, but cannot perform proper glycosylation, making them more suitable for production of antibody fragments. Product recovery and refolding may be a problem, and capital costs are also high.

Transgenic animals, including goats, cattle and chickens offer the advantage of lower material and product costs, and proper glycoform generation. Production levels can be increased by increasing the size of the herd, however the lead time for building up herds may be considerable, although less than that required to build physical plant facilities. Concerns over prions and viruses require careful consideration of hygiene standards.

Transgenic plants represent the final alternative, again with attendant advantages and disadvantages. Recognizing these limitations, Fiedler et al., (1997) tried to optimize the accumulation and stability of functionally active single chain Fv antibodies in transgenic tobacco plants. High accumulation of the two different scFv proteins in transgenic tobacco plants was only achieved by retention of the recombinant antibodies in the lumen of the endoplasmic reticulum (ER). A plant expression system where the scFv-proteins are targeted in the ER provides not only the highest accumulation level of active single chain Fv antibodies ever reported but also a short- or long-term storage of the foreign protein in the harvested plant material.

Application of these approaches could drive down costs even more than the optimistic predictions voiced by plant biotech company representatives. Since the theoretical potential is the lowest of any method, plants could in the future be the technology of choice. They have the capability to meet extremely high demand, greater than 500 kg/year. But the time to establish stocks may be substantial, and production sites may require special security.

5.2.2   Limitations of mammalian cell culture

CHO cells are approved by the FDA for most recombinant human glycoprotein production, since the glycosylation machinery is similar to the human system. However, CHO cells may not be adequate to satisfy long term industrial requirements for the production of antibodies. Other options include plasmacytoma cell lines such as the rat Y0 line whose natural glycosylation profile included the presence of bisecting GLcNAc residues. A further concern is the possibility that mutant clones may arise during extensive and continuous culture with the emergence and overgrowth of a sub-clone secreting structurally and functionally aberrant molecules. The reality of this concern is demonstrated by the isolation of multiple sub-clones of CHO cells expressing an altered profile of glycosyltransferases and secreting glycoproteins with unique glycoform profiles (Lee, et al., 2001).

Pilot studies, while they may provide information allowing optimization of growth conditions, may yield protocols too expensive to transfer into commercial production. Ideally, one would aim for a system that mimics in vivo conditions (homeostasis) as closely as possibly with the maintenance of nutrient concentration, oxygen tension and removal of metabolites.

A major consideration for the industry is the overall cost of production. An important element in its determination is downstream processing. Isolation and purification is simplified by the use of defined media and there has been a sustained development of serum free media with most companies adopting their own proprietary formulation. Large-scale production facilities have employed air-lifting fermenters of 10,000-20,000 L capacity. Cultures may be gradually expanded, moving to the next larger fermenter to allow exponential growth. At the end stage the cells exhaust the medium, die and their endogenous proteins are released following rupture of the cell membranes. Hollow fiber bioreactors have been used for research and intermediate scale production of glycoprotein, including antibodies to be used as *in vivo* therapeutics. This system does allow continuous exchange between the medium. However, the cells are not homogeneously dispersed throughout the cell compartment but grow in clumps of solid tissue. The result of these sub-optimal conditions is that mass transfer across such a tissue is curtailed and hence necrosis follows.

5.3   Total in vitro chemical synthesis of proteins and their glycosylation sites

Advances in carbohydrate chemistry, aided by recombinant glycosyltransferases, may permit synthetic construction of complex oligosaccharides. These could then be grafted onto recombinant proteins made in prokaryotic systems. At present, the Neose Company has the capacity to remodel glycoprotein in the range of grams. Currently, there are several efficient expression systems available that are capable of producing commercial scale quantities of enzymes required for *in vitro* glycosylation. Glycosyltransferases, such as sialyltransferases, galactosyltransferases and fucosyltransferases are expressed in *Aspergillis niger*, a GRAS (Generally Recognized As Safe) organism, as a fusion protein with a cleavage signal which can be easily removed. Until this technology is developed and expanded to industrial scales, animal cells will remain the first choice for the production of most human recombinant glycoprotein therapeutics.

REFERENCES

Abiko, Y. 2000. Passive immunization against dental caries and periodontic disease: development of recombinant and human monoclonal antibodies. *Crit Rev Oral Biol Med* 11(2):140-158.

Andersen, D. C., Goochee, C. F., Cooper, G. and Weitzhandler, M. 1994. Monosaccharide and oligosaccharide analysis of isoelectric focusing-separated and blotted granulocyte colony-stimulating factor glycoforms using high-pH anion-exchange chromatography with pulsed amperometric detection. Glycobiology 4(4):459-467.

Bernstein, R.E. 1987. Nonenzymatically glycosylated proteins. *Adv Clin Chem* 26:1-78.

Borrebaeck, C. K., Malmborg, A. C. and Ohlin, M. 1993. Does endogenous glycosylation prevent the use of mouse monoclonal antibodies as cancer therapeutics? *Immunol Today* 14(10): 477-479.

Borys, M.C., Linzer, D.I., Papoutsakis, E.T. 1994. Cell aggregation in a Chinese hamster ovary cell microcarrier culture affects the expression rate and N-linked glycosylation of recombinant mouse placental lactogen-1. *Ann N Y Acad Sci* 745:360-371.

Chargelegue, D., Vine, N. D., van Dolleweerd, C. J., Drake, P. M. and Ma, J. K. 2000. A murine monoclonal antibody produced in transgenic plants with plant-specific glycans is not immunogenic in mice. *Transgenic Res* 9(3): 187-194.

Choi, B. K., Bleck, G. T. and Jimenez-Flores, R. 2001. Cation-exchange purification of mutagenized bovine beta-casein expressed in transgenic mouse milk: its putative Asn68-linked glycan is heterogeneous. *J Dairy Sci* 84(1):44-49.

Das, R., and Morrow, K. J. 2002. *Antibody Engineering: Technologies, Applications and Business Opportunities Report 9038*. D&MD Reports. Westborough, MA.

Dwek, R. A. 1995. Glycobiology: more functions for oligosaccharides. *Science* 269(5228):1234-1235.

Fiedler, U., Phillips, J., Artsaenko, O. and Conrad, U. 1997. Optimization of scFv antibody production in transgenic plants. *Immunotechnology*3(3):205-216.

Gauny, S. S., Andya, J., Thomson, J., Young, J. D. and Winkelhake, J.L. 1991. Effect of production method on the systemic clearance rate of a human monoclonal antibody in the rat. *Hum Antibodies Hybridomas* 2(1): 33-38

Gillies, S.D., Morrison, S.L., Oi, V.T., Tonegawa, S. 1983. A tissue-specific transcription enhancer element is located in the major intron of a rearranged immunoglobulin heavy chain gene. *Cell* 33(3): 717-728.

Hamadeh, R. M., Jarvis, G. A., Zhou, P., Cotleur, A. C. and Griffiss, J. M. 1996. Bacterial enzymes can add galactose alpha 1,3 to human erythrocytes and creates a senescence-associated epitope. *Infect Immun* 64(2): 528-34.

Hayter, P. M., Curling, E. M., Gould M. L., Baines, A. J., Jenkins, N., Salmon, I., Strange, P. G., and Bull, A. T. 1993. The effect of dilution rate on CHO cell physiology and recombinant interferon γ production in glucose limited chemostat culture. *Biotechnol Bioengineer* 42: 1077-1085.

Hein, M. B., Tang, Y., McLeod, D.A., Janda, K. D.and Hiatt, A. 1991. Evaluation of immunoglobulins from plant cells. *Biotechnol Prog* 7(5):455-61

Hiatt, A. 1992. Monoclonal antibody engineering in plants. FEBS Lett. 307(1): 71-75.

Jefferis, R. and Lund, J. 1997. Glycosylation of antibody molecules: structure and functional significance. *Chem. Immnol* 65:111-128

Jefferis, R., Takahashi, N., Lund, J., Tyler, R., Hindley, S. 1992. Does an antibody molecule act as a template directing (determining) its glycosylation? *Biochem Soc Trans.* 20(2): 228S.

Jenkins, N. Growth factors. 1992. In: *Mammalian Cell Biotechnology, A Practical Approach* (Butler, M. ed). pp 39-55. Oxford University Press. Oxford, UK.

Jenkins, N. and Curling, E. M. 1994. Glycosylation of recombinant proteins: problems and prospects. *Enzyme Microb Technol* **16**(5): 354-364.

Jenkins, N., Parekh, R. B., and James, D. C. 1996. Getting the glycosylation right: implications for the biotechnology industry. *Nat Biotechnol* **14**(8): 975-981.

Johnson, P. M., Watkins, J., Scopes, P. M. and Tracey, B. M. 1974. Differences in serum IgG structure in health and rheumatoid disease. Circular dichroism studies. *Ann Rheum Dis* **33**(4): 366-370.

Kornfeld, R., Kornfeld, S. 1985. Assembly of asparagine-linked oligosaccharides. *Annu Rev Biochem* **54**: 631-664.

Koyama, J., Morita, I., Kawanishi, K., Tagahara, K., Kobayashi, N. 2003. Capillary Electrophoresis for Simultaneous Determination of Emodin, Chrysophanol, and Their 8-beta-D-Glucosides. *Chem Pharm Bull (Tokyo)* **51**(4): 418-420.

Kumar, M., Mishra, N. and Upreti, R. K. 2003. A novel membrane glycoprotein of Escherichia coli. *J Basic Microbiol* **43**(1): 28-35.

Kumpel, B. M., Rademacher, T. W., Rook, G. A., Williams, P. J. and Wilson, I. B. 1994. Galactosylation of human IgG monoclonal anti-D produced by EBV-transformed B-lymphoblastoid cell lines is dependent on culture method and affects Fc receptor-mediated functional activity. *Hum Antibodies Hybridomas* **5**(3-4): 143-151.

Kunkel, J.P., Jan, D.C., Butler, M., Jamieson, J.C. 2000. Comparisons of the glycosylation of a monoclonal antibody produced under nominally identical cell culture conditions in two different bioreactors. *Biotechnol Prog* **16**(3): 462-470.

Lapuk, V. A., Timofeev, V. P., Tchukchrova, A. I., Khatiashvili, N. M. and Kiseleva, T. M. 1984. Some peculiarities of the dynamics of the immunoglobulin M structure. *J Biomol Struct Dyn* **2**(1): 63-76.

Lee, E. U., Roth, J. and Paulson, J. C. 1989. Alteration of terminal glycosylation sequences on N-linked oligosaccharides of Chinese hamster ovary cells by expression of beta-galactoside alpha 2,6-sialyltransferase. *J Biol Chem* **264**(23): 13848-13855.

Lee, J., Sundaram, S., Shaper, N. L., Raju, T. S. and Stanley, P. 2001. Chinese hamster ovary (CHO) cells may express six beta 4-galactosyltransferases (beta 4GalTs). Consequences of the loss of functional beta 4GalT-1, beta 4GalT-6, or both in CHO glycosylation mutants. *J Biol Chem* **276**(17): 13924-13934.

Leibiger, H., Hansen, A., Schoenherr, G., Seifert, M., Wustner, D., Stigler, R. and Marx, U. 1995. Glycosylation analysis of a polyreactive human monoclonal IgG antibody derived from a human-mouse heterohybridoma. *Mol Immunol* **32**(8): 595-602.

Lee, E. U., Roth, J. and Paulson, J. C. 1989. Alteration of terminal glycosylation sequences on N-linked oligosaccharides of Chinese hamster ovary cells by expression of beta-galactosidase alpha 2,6-sialyltransferase. J Biol Chem **264**(23): 13848-13855.

Leibiger, H., Wustner, D., Stigler, R.D., Marx, U. 1999. Variable domain-linked oligosaccharides of a human monoclonal IgG: structure and influence on antigen binding. *Biochem J 338* (Pt 2): 529-538.

Lifely, M. R., Hale, C., Boyce, S., Keen, M. J. and Phillips, J. 1995. Glycosylation and biological activity of CAMPATH-1H expressed in different cell lines and grown under different culture conditions. *Glycobiology* **5**(8): 813-822.

Lund, J., Takahashi, N., Nakagawa, H., Goodall, M., Bentley, T., Hindley, S.A., Tyler, R., Jefferis, R. 1993. Control of IgG/Fc glycosylation: a comparison of oligosaccharides from chimeric human/mouse and mouse subclass immunoglobulin Gs. *Mol Immunol* **30**(8):741-748.

Ma, J.K., Hiatt, A., Hein, M., Vine, N.D., Wang, F., Stabila, P., van Dolleweerd, C., Mostov, K., Lehner, T. 1995. Generation and assembly of secretory antibodies in plants. *Science* **268**(5211): 716-719.

Marx, U. 1998. Membrane-based cell culture technologies: a scientifically and economically satisfactory alternative to malignant ascites production for monoclonal antibodies. *Res Immunol* **149**(6): 557-559.

Monica, T. J., Goochee, C. F. and Maiorella, B. L. 1993. Comparative biochemical characterization of a human IgM produced in both ascites and in vitro cell culture. *Biotechnology* 11(4): 512-515.

Monica, T. J., Williams, S.B., Goochee, C.F., Maiorella, B.L. 1995. Characterization of the glycosylation of a human IgM produced by a human-mouse hybridoma. *Glycobiology* 5(2): 175-185.

Nakao, H., Nishikawa, A., Karasuno, T., Nishiura, T., Iida, M., Kanayama, Y., Yonezawa, T., Tarui, S., Taniguchi, N. 1990. n-butyrate reduces the expression of beta-galactoside alpha 2,6-sialyltransferase in Hep G2 cells. *Biochem Biophys Res Commun* 172(3): 1260-1266.

Patel, T.P., Parekh, R.B., Moellering, B.J., Prior, C.P. 1992 Different culture methods lead to differences in glycosylation of a murine IgG monoclonal antibody. *Biochem J* 285(Pt 3): 839-845.

Potter, M. and Lieberman, R. 1970. Common individual antigenic determinants in five of eight BALB-c IgA myeloma proteins that bind phosphoryl choline. J Exp Med 132(4): 737-751.

Rabina, J., Maki, M., Savilahti, E.M., Jarvinen, N., Penttila, L. and Renkonen, R. 2001. Analysis of nucleotide sugars from cell lysates by ion-pair solid-phase extraction and reversed-phase high-performance liquid chromatography. *Glycoconj J* 18(10): 799-805.

Raju, T. S., Briggs, J. B., Chamow, S. M., Winkler, M. E., and Jones, A. J. S. 2001. Glycoengineering of Therapeutic Glycoproteins: In vitro galactosylation and sialylation of glycoproteins with terminal *N*-Acetylglucosamine and galactose residues. *Biochemistry* 40(30): 8868-8876.

Robbe, C., Capon, C., Flahaut, C. and Michalski, J.C. 2003. Microscale analysis of mucin-type O-glycans by a coordinated and mass spectrometry approach. *Electrophoresis* 24(4): 611-621.

Rudd, P. M., Leatherbarrow, R. J., Rademacher, T. W., Dwek, R.A. 1991. Diversification of the IgG molecule by oligosaccharides. *Mol Immuno* l28(12):1369-1378.

Rudisser, S., Jahnke W. 2002. NMR and in silico screening. Comb Chem High Throughput Screen 5(8):591-603.

Schenerman, M. A., Hope, J. N., Kletke, C., Singh, J. K., Kimura, R., Tsao, E. I. and Folena-Wasserman G. 1999. Comparability testing of a humanized monoclonal antibody (Synagis) to support cell line stability, process validation, and scale-up for manufacturing. *Biologicals* 27(3): 203-215.

Shah, S., Lance, P., Smith, T. J., Berenson, C. S., Cohen, S. A., Horvath, P. J., Lau, J. T. and Baumann, H. 1992. n-butyrate reduces the expression of beta-galactoside alpha 2,6-sialyltransferase in Hep G2 cells. *J Biol Chem* 267(15): 10652-10658.

Silverman, H.S., Sutton-Smith, M., McDermott, K., Heal, P., Leir, S.H., Morris, H.R., Hollingsworth, M.A., Dell, A., Harris, A. 2003. The contribution of tandem repeat number to the O-Glycosylation of mucins. Glycobiology 13(4): 265-277.

Stanfield, R. L., Fieser, T. M., Lerner, R. A. and Wilson, I. 1990. A Crystal structures of an antibody to a peptide and its complex with peptide antigen at 2.8 A. *Science* 248(4956): 712-719.

Stanley, P. 1992. Glycosylation Engineering. *Glycobiology* 2(2): 99-107.

Uesson, M., Hansson, U.B. 1982. Circular dichroism of immune complexes, IgG and Fab gamma with unique antigenic determinants from rheumatoid serum. *Scand J Immunol* 16(3): 249-256.

Umana, P., Jean-Mairet, J., Moudry, R, Amstutz, H., Bailey, J. E. 1999. Engineered glycoforms of an antineuroblastoma IgG1 with optimized antibody-dependent cellular cytotoxic activity. *Nat Biotechnol* 17(2): 176-180.

Van Berkel, P. H., Welling, M. M., Geerts, M., van Veen, H. A., Ravensbergen, B., Salaheddine, M., Pauwels, E. K., Pieper, F., Nuijens, J. H. and Nibbering, P. H. 2002. Large scale production of recombinant human lactoferrin in the milk of transgenic cows. *Nat Biotechnol* 20(5): 484-487.

Wacker. M., Linton, .D, Hitchen, P. G., Nita-Lazar, M., Haslam, S. M., North, S. J., Panico, M., Morris, H. R., Dell, A., Wren, B. W. and Aebi, M. 2002. N-linked glycosylation in Campylobacter jejuni and its functional transfer into E. coli. *Science* **298**(5599):1790-1793.

Wang, F., Nakouzi, A., Hogue Angeletti, R. and Casadevall, A. 2003. Site-specific characterization of the N-linked oligosaccharides of a murine immunoglobulin M by high-performance liquid chromatography/ electrospray mass spectrometry. *Anal Biochem.***314**(2):266-280.

Weikert, S., Papac, D., Briggs, J., Cowfer, D., Tom, S., Gawlitzek, M., Lofgren, J., Mehta, S., Chisholm· V., Modi, N., Eppler, S., Carroll, K., Chamow, S., Peers, D., Berman, P. & L. Krummen. 1999. Engineering Chinese hamster ovary cells to maximize sialic acid content of recombinant glycoproteins. *Nature Biotechnology.* **17**: 1116 –1121.

Wormald, M. R., Rudd, P. M., Harvey, D. J., Chang, S. C., Scragg, I. G. and Dwek, R. A.. 1997. Variations in oligosaccharide-protein interactions in immunoglobulin G determine the site-specific glycosylation profiles and modulate the dynamic motion of the Fc oligosaccharides. *Biochemistry* **36**(6): 1370-1380.

Yoo, E. M., Koteswara, R., Chintalacharuvu, M. L. and Morrison, S. L. 2002. Myeloma expression systems. *J. Immun Methods* **261**(1-2): 1-20.

Youings, A., Chang, S. C., Dwek, R. A. and Scragg, I. G. 1996. Site-specific glycosylation of human immunoglobulin G is altered in four rheumatoid arthritis patients. *Biochem J* **314**(2): 621-630.

Zeitlin, L., Olmsted, S. S., Moench, T. R., Co M. S., Martinell, B. J., Paradkar V. M., Russell, D.R., Queen, C., Cone, R.A. and Whaley, K. J. 1998. A humanized monoclonal antibody produced in transgenic plants for immunoprotection of the vagina against genital herpes. *Nat Biotechno* **16**(13):1361-1364.

Chapter 4

APPROACHES TO DEVISE ANTIBODY PURIFICATION PROCESSES BY CHROMATOGRAPHY

Egisto Boschetti
Ciphergen Biosystems – Biosepra, 48, Avenue des Genottes, Cergy, France

1.   INTRODUCTION

Monoclonal antibodies and more largely immunoglobulins along with all their fragments and engineered forms represent today the largest class of produced and purified protein in number and quantity. New potential applications of antibodies in their native form or various engineered constructs actually continue to stimulate therapeutic areas. Expected high dosage levels imply that their purity has to meet stringent requirements. It means also that the production cost per dose compared to other therapeutic biomolecules has to be kept low. To achieve these goals it is anticipated that effective, low cost productions and purification strategies will be put in place.

The purification of antibodies has a story that commenced with the separation of proteins several decades ago. Many approaches have been described involving precipitation with a variety of chemical agents, electrophoresis-based fractionations, membrane methodologies and liquid chromatography. The latter probably represents the most largely used approach as a result of the easy to be implemented, the capability to modulate on the selectivity and finally the level of purity that can be achieved. Interestingly a large number of specific chromatographic sorbents has been developed for the purpose, a peculiar situation that has no equivalent in the bioseparation world.

Although various purification principles for antibodies have been developed, the most commonly used technique is to selectively adsorb them on Protein A sorbents from very crude feedstocks [Ey, 1978; Duffy, 1989]. The high selectivity of Protein A for the Fc fragment facilitates the separation of antibodies; however, this approach is associated with high costs and various practical complications [Fuglistaller, 1989; Godfrey, 1993]. Alternatives to Protein A chromatography are affinity or pseudo-affinity sorbents that provide a good compromise between selectivity and cost. Thiophilic chromatography [Belew, 1987; Boschetti, 2001a] and bio-mimetic affinity chromatography [Li,1998; Palombo, 1998] have been developed and applied to achieve this objective. Effectively enough these methods eliminate some specific drawbacks related to Protein A chromatography; nevertheless they are still limited due to the necessity to work either in the presence of highly concentrated lyotropic salts, the necessity to design relatively complicated chemically structured ligands or even to change conditions of pH and ionic strength prior the adsorption step. Other sorbents or methods have been developed for antibody separation: peptodomimetic ligands [Guerrier, 1998; Lihme, 1997; Palombo, 1998], arenophilic sorbents [Ngo, 1994], thiophilic aromatic solid phases [Scholz, 1998a] and histidine based matrix [El-Kak, 1992]. All these mentioned methods are based on different adsorption/desorption principles.

Antibodies are a homogeneous family of proteins with very different biochemical properties; they have in common several well-known highly conserved properties such as the presence of loci with clusters of histidine, large hydrophobic regions, and well-determined glycosylated sites. This is the main reason why various strategies have been employed to design solid phases for their separation [for a whole review see Boschetti, 2000].

In spite of these peculiar properties, ion exchange chromatography remains one of the most popular methods for antibody separation from the very first step. Strong and weak cation [Carlsson, 1985; Necina, 1998] and anion [Duffy, 1989] exchange chromatography procedures have been described and are still in use.

Optimal conditions of protein adsorption and desorption, have been demonstrated to be greatly dependent not only on characteristics of antibodies, but also on the number and amount of foreign proteins. Environmental pH and ionic strength are both critical for an efficient antibody capture. When the separation process uses more than one column the coherence between buffers and the right sequence of columns must also to be established in an efficient way. In this situation, chromatographic conditions need to be properly defined every time the maximal enrichment of the antibody from a complex mixture is desired.

Throughout this chapter essential separation methods for antibody purifications are described with respect to chromatography sorbents. Although the review is far from exhaustive, it discusses technologies that either are or will become the most relevant approaches in this domain, because of their effectiveness and their large scale possible exploitation. After the description of separation methods a section is devoted to the design of a separation process. This notion is in fact one of most obscure and controversial steps for process design where the goal is to reach an optimal level in terms of recovery, robustness and cost.

2. Ion exchange chromatography: role, strengths and weaknesses

Ion exchange is extensively applied to antibody separation. Separation selectivity and efficiency depend on a number of factors, which have been studied in depth in theory and practice. A large variety of resins for different applications has been described and is commercially available.

Ion-exchangers are classified into four categories according to their electrical charge and the shape of the titration curve; weak and strong cation and weak and strong anion exchangers. Concepts and mechanisms of action of modern ion exchangers have been extensively described [see Boschetti, 2002a for review].

For the adsorption of antibodies virtually all ion exchangers compatible with protein separation can be used. Anion exchangers have been used extensively for the isolation of polyclonal IgG from human plasma and from different mammals in a single step with a high degree of purity [Danielsson, 1988; Chen, 1988].

They have also been used for the isolation of isoforms of monoclonal IgG after optimization of adsorption and elution conditions to fit with the isoelectric point properties of the antibody [McLaren, 1994].

Antibodies are actually very diverse in their isoelectric point, which can be between 4 to 9. This is why isoelectric point of the antibody is a parameter to consider for an appropriate choice of an ion exchanger and of a buffer. However, the net charge conferred by amino acid composition does not take in consideration clusters of ionisable groups on the surface of the protein that play a role in the interaction with solid surfaces. Moreover the isoelectric point determination is obviously ineffective for polyclonal antibodies. An antibody should adsorb on an anion exchanger at pH value above its pI and to a cation exchanger below its pI. This rule is however valid only at low conductivity conditions, because the presence of small ions in the running buffer prevents antibody adsorption by competition.

Sufficient adsorption of antibodies on cation exchange resins is generally reached in running buffers with low ionic strength, which is equivalent to a conductivity of 10 mS/cm or lower at a pH between 4 and 6. At a pH above 8 and low ionic strength, sufficient adsorption is reached for an anion exchanger. Desorption at laboratory scale is effected by a linear sodium chloride gradient or by a pH gradient or both. The peak position in linear gradient elution can be used to determine the required salt concentration for stepwise elution, which is preferred at both pilot and industrial scale.

Ion exchange chromatography can be applied to virtually all monoclonal antibody separation from different classes, species and feedstocks. Due to the diversity of antibodies and impurities to remove adsorption and elution conditions must be empirically determined case-by-case. Since it is not possible to predict the adsorption behaviour on ion-exchangers from the amino acid sequence, alternative methods have been designed as described on following sections.

Most of the time physicochemical properties of crude feedstocks are not compatible with a direct adsorption of antibodies on ion exchangers; therefore the ionic strength and or pH must be modified significantly. In practice the actual salt concentration depends on the net charge of the antibody and the charge density of the ion-exchanger. The easiest way to adsorb an antibody on an ion exchange resin is to dilute the feedstock to lower the conductivity to about 5 mS/cm. This is not always practical particularly when dealing with large volumes to process. Additionally if the antibody concentration is below certain limits, a proper adsorption on the resin does not occur. Diafiltration followed by a concentration step, whenever appropriate, are additional operations to adjust the properties of the feedstock to be suited for adsorption on an ion exchange resin [Jiskoot, 1989].

To circumvent feedstock dilution, special cation exchangers with high charge density are used for antibody capture. Representatives of highly substituted ion exchangers are, CM Ceramic HyperD, CM HyperZ and Sepharose XL. They carry 300-400 µmols of carboxyl groups per ml of packed resin. Using these resins, specific studies demonstrated the possibility to efficiently adsorb antibodies directly from crude feed streams with conductivities as high as 22 mS/cm.

Binding capacities of such sorbents are higher than 60 mg/ml in physiological conditions. pH for adsorption, must nevertheless to be adjusted according to the individual property of the antibody, but pH should be always in the range of 4.2 and 4.8.

The purity of antibodies that can be reached by ion exchange chromatography in a single pass is 40-98%. This depends on the choice of the ion exchanger, and on the nature of feedstock carrying protein impurities.

Ion-exchange chromatography can be used as a capture step at the initial stage of antibody separation and then be followed by one or two additional chromatography steps to remove contaminants.

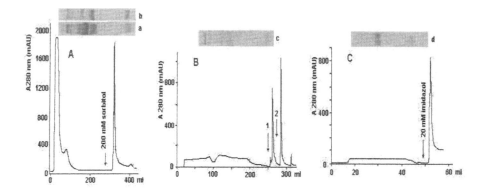

Figure 4.1. Three-step antibody separation from bovine serum using Boronate HyperCel (A), Q HyperZ (B) and IMAC HyperCel (C). Crude serum was injected in the first column in physiological conditions and then glycoproteins desorbed with sorbitol. This fraction was directly loaded in the second column and desorption of proteins was performed using a 75 mM (1) and 150 mM (2) sodium chloride solution at pH 8. Fraction 1 was then loaded on Cu^{++} IMAC column from which IgG were eluted using a 20 mM imidazol solution at pH 7. Inserts represent SDS electrophoresis results. a: crude bovine serum; b: IgG-rich boronate fraction; c: IgG-rich Q column fraction; d: pure IgG from IMAC column.

Alternatively ion exchange chromatography can be advantageously used for the separation of impurities coming from an affinity capture. The nature of the ion exchanger is chosen not only by the best separation properties, but also for the direct compatibility with the preceding column.

Figure 1 illustrates a practical example of the use of an anion exchanger after antibody capture to reduce the complexity.

Asdorption of polyclonal antibodies from bovine serum is first accomplished on a boronate sorbent. Glycoproteins including IgG are thus adsorbed on the column leaving in the flowthrough a large amount of proteins, among them, albumin. Immunoglobulins are desorbed quite selectively by a solution of sorbitol. The semicrude collected protein fraction is separated by ion exchange in classical conditions. Collected IgG under a salt gradient are then polished using an IMAC sorbent chelated with copper. This three-step separation resulted effectively into a pure IgG fraction. Buffers used were compatible from column to column.

Since ion exchangers cannot be used at neutral pH, it should be noticed that anion exchangers (typically used at pH around 8) may induce the activation of proteases such as trypsin-like proteases as well as plasmin and kallikrein when traces are present in the feedstock.

3.   PSEUDO-AFFINITY VERSUS BIO-AFFINITY

It is generally admitted that affinity chromatography involves solid phase sorbents on which bio-specific ligands against the protein to separate are chemically attached. The construct is then used for the specific adsorption of the target protein in physiological conditions from a very crude feedstock. The column is then washed to remove foreign species and the protein of interest desorbed by selected means.

The key for the preparation of an affinity sorbent is the selection of the appropriate ligand, the adapted immobilization chemistry and the linker or spacer arm.

Modelling approaches of affinity interactions are well known; the specificity of the interaction is a probabilistic term that is dependent on the law of mass action between two molecular species [Boschetti, 2000].

Solid phase material, chemical activation, principle of covalent link for the bio-specific ligand and conditions of adsorption and desorption are extensively described [Carlsson, 1988].

3.1   Bio-affinity chromatography

Bio-specific affinity chromatography for antibody separation is characterized by three main base concepts: (i) antibody-antibody based affinity recognition, (ii) antigen-antibody affinity interaction and (iii) protein A-antibody (and related proteins) specific adsorption.

The use of specific antibodies as immobilized affinity ligands constitutes an effective way to selectively purify monoclonal as well as polyclonal antibodies. Anti-immunoglobulins are chemically coupled on a solid phase chromatographic matrix and used as an affinity sorbent. An advantage of this approach is its extreme specificity. Additionally the antibody ligand can be chosen as a function of its affinity constant so as elution conditions remains mild for a minimum denaturation of the antibody to be separated.

The adsorption phase is performed in physiological conditions of pH and ionic strength; elution of antibodies is generally obtained by acidic deforming buffers such as 0.2 M glycine-HCl, pH 2-3.

Immunoaffinity chromatography using an antibody as the ligand is, however, so specific that it is necessary to design a sorbent each time a new antibody is to be separated. This implies the production of a specific antibody ligand, its purification and then its immobilization on a solid matrix. Overall the process is a relatively expensive and has applications restricted to laboratory scale. For a more broad applicability, antibody ligands against heavy or light chains can be used to purify antibodies of the same group [Bazin, 1984a; Bazin, 1984b].

Typical molecules that are specifically recognized by antibodies are antigens; therefore the immobilization of an antigen (protein or hapten) on a chromatographic matrix constitutes a mean to selectively purify antibodies. For the implementation of such an approach, the first requirement is the availability of the antigen prior its chemical immobilization on a solid matrix. For small sized antigen molecules, a spacer arm may be required in order to ensure accessibility to the active site of the antibody [Mohan, 1997].

The most common bio-affinity technique to separate antibodies is based on the use of Protein A and related bacterial proteinaceous ligands.

Table 4.1: Antibodies that do not interact with Protein A

Specie	Type of antibody	Interaction
Human	IgG3, IgA, IgM	Weak interaction
Mouse	IGM	No interaction
Rat	IgG2a, IgG2b, IgM	No interaction
Goat, Sheep, Mouse	IgG1	Weak interaction
Goat, Sheep, Rabbit	IgM	No interaction
Chicken	IgY	No interaction

Protein A is a cell wall constituent of *Staphylococcus aureus* with high specificity for Fc fragment of many IgG antibodies. This biomolecule is constituted of a single polypeptide chain with a C-terminus related to a trans-membrane domain and five homologous IgG-binding regions [Moks, 1986]. Its molecular mass is 41,000 Daltons and its isoelectric point is about 5.

Protein A ligand has been grafted to many solid porous chromatographic supports such as agarose, dextran beads, silica, HyperD and others. The primary binding site of Protein A is the Fc fragment of IgG at the junctures of CH2 and CH3 domains. Its specificity is very high, however it does not interact with all IgG antibodies (see Table 4.1 and Figure 4.2).

The advantage of using Protein A is that most of the time prediction of separation of antibodies is demonstrated and conditions of separation of impurities can be done using predetermined pHs and ionic strengths with no need of optimization. The adsorption phase is also compatible with most types of feedstocks, with no necessity to dilute, concentrate or to use additives. Although binding of IgG onto Protein A resins generally takes place in physiological conditions, the presence of polyethylene glycols, glycine buffers at high pHs and high ionic strength enhances the interaction. Interaction is complex, but one of dominant contribution is hydrophobic association.

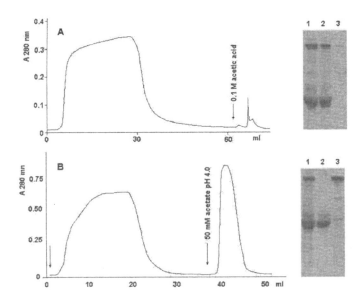

Figure 4.2. Comparative separation of rat monoclonal antibodies from hybridoma cell culture supernatant in the presence of 10% fetal bovine serum on Protein A Ceramic HyperD (A) and MEP HyperCel (B). Loading conditions were similar for both columns: direct injection of crude supernatant in physiological conditions. Elution was accomplished by using respectively 0.1 M acetic acid, pH 3 or 50 mM acetate buffer, pH 4. As shown in inserts, Protein A sorbent was unable to capture properly rat antibodies (see also Table 1): most of the antibody was found in the flowthrough (A2). Virtually no antibody was found in the acetic acid fraction (A3). Conversely MEP HyperCel captured all antibodies (no antibody found in the flowthrough fraction B2), which were thus collected by elution with acetate buffer (B3). Contaminants in trace amount were albumin and a second unidentified protein. Lanes 1 of both electrophoresis analysis represent initial crude samples.

Elution of antibodies from Protein A can be accomplished using acidic pH in the region of 2.5-3. When the adsorption is performed at alkaline pH and high ionic strength, for instance when adsorbing mouse IgG1, the elution can be obtained just by lowering the ionic strength at a pH close to 5-6. Binding capacity for antibodies is also satisfactory for preparative purposes.

These advantages are unfortunately counterbalanced by a number of disadvantages at different levels. Biologically speaking the association of Protein A with Fc fragment of IgG affects somewhat the local structure of the antibody, destabilizing the structure of carbohydrate moiety with consequent altered susceptibility to proteolytic attack. This interaction can also partially alter antibody effector functions. Additionally, the necessity to use acidic conditions to desorb captured antibodies contributes to aggregation and some denaturation for acidic-sensitive antibodies.

As a protein based ligand, Protein A cannot be cleaned in the presence of caustic solutions as it is the case for chemical ligands; this situation renders the use of protein A less practical in term of sanitization and longevity. Although it is relatively stable, Protein A can be degraded with consequent leakage of fragments that may contaminate the antibody production. Actually Protein A leakage (as whole and/or under proteolysis fragments) is one of the most serious arguments that limit its use [Fuglistaller, 1989; Godfrey, 1993; Peng, 1986]. Cost of Protein A resins is also prohibitively high: this necessitates specific care to maintain the column as long as possible for multiple uses.

In spite of all the described limitations, Protein A sorbents are the most popular means to adsorb specifically antibodies for small and large scale applications.

Table 4. 2: Protein with affinity for antibodies

Protein ligand	Origin	Specificity	Type of antibody
Protein A	*Staphylococcus a.*	Fc fragment	Most of IgG
Protein G	Streptococci (G, C)	Fc	All IgG
Protein L	*Peptococcus m.*	K chains	IgM, IgG
Protein P	*Clostridium p.*	K chains	IgM
Protein ARP	A streptococci	Fc	IgA
Concanavalin A	*Concanavalia e.*	Glycosylated region	IgG, IgM, IgA
Jacalin	*Artrocarpus h.*	Glycosylated region	IgA, IgE
RCA-2	*Ricinus c.*	Glycosylated region	IgD
LCA	*Lens c.*	Glycosylated region	IgG, IgM
GNA	*Galanthus n.*	Glycosylated region	IgM

A number of other microbial proteins are known for the separation of antibodies (see Table 4.2). One of them is Protein G [Akerstrom1986]. Similarly to Protein A, it is also composed of a single polypeptide chain with binding domains for IgG. Recombinant versions of Protein G have been engineered to remove selected undesired domains but keeping intact the IgG binding region. In spite of similar specificity for antibodies, binding sites for IgG are composed of sequences that are different from those for Protein A specificity. This is why the applicability spectrum of Protein G is different in term of specificity for antibodies classes, subclasses and species. Among other bacterial protein ligands for antibodies Protein L from *Peptostreptococcus magnus* deserves to be mentioned. It binds specifically to the variable domain of immunoglobulin light chain without interfering with the antigen binding site [Nilson, 1993]. It binds all classes of human antibodies comprising kappa light chains.

3.2   Synthetic ligands for antibody adsorption

Pseudo-affinity methods use ligands having an affinity for antibodies similar to the bio-affinity partner. The interaction generally involves more than one molecular association parameter; among them are ionic interactions, hydrophobic associations and other minor molecular forces.

In the last few years a number of chemical structures have been described with the objective to circumvent the drawbacks of Protein A mentioned above; some of them are actually called "Protein A mimetic ligands".

Some described Protein A mimetic ligand are based on a rational approach in understanding the structures of natural docking domains between the B domain of Protein A and the Fc fragment of IgG. Studies in this field generated several ligand candidates with affinity for immunoglobulins G [Li, 1998; Teng, 1999; Teng, 2000].

Since the interaction appeared to be predominantly hydrophobic and supported by some hydrogen bonding effects, the structures studied focused around phenylalanine, tyrosine and isoleucine residues. These aminoacids were attached to a trichlorotriazine ring in different proportions and the various structures obtained were studied for their affinity for IgG.

Measured affinity constant obtained with these ligands where in the range of 10^2 - 10^4 compared to 1.4×10^7 for Protein A. Described purity of IgG from human plasma evaluated by SDS PAGE was reported to be in the range of 50 to 98 % when adsorption of IgG from a crude extract occurred in physiological conditions and elution was performed by lowering the pH to 3.8 and below.

In other reports a series of peptides with the ability to interact with immunoglobulins were described and have been used as affinity chromatography ligand [Guerrier, 1998; Fassina, 1998; Fassina, 2001]. These peptide structures resulted from a combinatorial peptide library screening methodology and were identified by their ability to make complexes with IgG that were displaced by the addition of Protein A. As for the previous described peptidomimetic ligands, they do not distinguish classes of antibodies. Binding capacity of sorbents made with these peptide ligands were reported to be close to 15 mg per ml of resin.

The separation of immunoglobulins is performed by adsorbing the material in 100 mM phosphate buffer and after a washing step immunoglobulins are desorbed by increasing the pH to 8-8.5 with carbonate or borate buffer. Similar results have also been recently published with a synthetic ligand able to mimic Protein A in the recognition of Fc portion of antibodies [Fassina, 1998]. Ligand specificity is broader than Protein A since IgG, IgA, IgM, IgE and IgY were all interacting with no specific discrimination. Elution was effective either at acidic pH (e.g. acetic acid) or using a sodium bicarbonate buffer pH 9. Purity checked by SDS-PAGE was higher than 90 % under the described conditions with a binding capacity that could reach up to 25 mg/ml of resin.

Another Protein A mimetic synthetic molecule was recently described [Lihme, 1997]. The nature of the ligand was not disclosed but its performance was reported as able to bind a large variety of immunoglobulins G and M from different animal species. In typical experiments binding capacity was in the range of 1.2 to 11.5 mg per ml of resin at pH 5.1; purity of immunoglobulins was in the range of 35 to 99 % and the recovery of 90-98 %. The use of sodium lauroyl sarcosinate was mentioned as a mean to avoid non specific binding.

Among the affinity related methods described for the separation of antibodies are sorbents carrying aza-arenophilic ligands [Ngo, 1992; Ngo, 1994] and immobilized histidine on agarose beads by means of aminohexyl spacer arm [El-Kak, 1992].

More recently a technique called hydrophobic charge induction chromatography was described [Boschetti, 2002b]. It is based on the use of a synthetic ligands associating hydrophobic properties for the adsorption of immunoglobulins, a heterocyclic structure and thiophilicity for antibody specificity, and ionisable groups to enhance the dissociation mechanism when changing the pH. This method is today extensively used for antibody purification at small and large scale.

Ligands designed for this technique are composed of a hydrophobic tail and of an ionizable head. They are covalently immobilized on matrices through their tail region by means of ether or thioether bonds.

The density of the ligand of the matrix is high so as to obtain IgG adsorption in physiological conditions of pH and of ionic strength. This approach seems much more acceptable to any other pseudo-affinity techniques because of a number of intrinsic benefits. Binding capacity is particularly high, specificity for antibody is high, the resin can be cleaned in very stringent conditions with no degradation, and resin and exploitation costs are fully affordable for small and compatible for large scale applications. This sorbent does not discriminate antibody classes or species.

The integral structure of the ligand is described as crucial for the specificity [Boschetti, 2001b]. Any minor change induces modifications in binding capacity or modifications of selectivity.

Hydrophobic charge induction chromatography is currently used for the separation of a number of immunoglobulins such as monoclonal antibodies from ascites fluid and cell culture supernatants, from bovine colostrum, cheese whey and from egg yolk.

Typically the adsorption phase is made without pH or ionic strength adjustment; the column is then washed with a 50 mM Tris buffer, pH 8 or a phosphate buffered saline. Desorption of albumin traces when present in the feedstock is washed out by water or sodium caprylate solution. Desorption of antibodies takes place by lowering the pH to 4 or below with low ionic strength buffers. Co-adsorption of albumin traces depends on the column saturation; when the column is highly loaded or in overloading conditions, albumin is displaced by IgG with resulting better purity for antibody. This approach obviates the use of an intermediate wash with water or sodium caprylate.

Variations of these conditions can be made during the adsorption phase to prevent capture of undesired impurities.

Elutions can also be modulated by using different buffers at acidic pH, such as acetate or citrate buffers. The higher the ionic strength of the buffer the lower the pH for a complete elution of antibodies. Purity for antibodies may be improved by pH elution step gradients according to the property of the antibody.

In a similar domain of ligand design, another structure is proposed for the capture of antibodies in lieu of Protein A. This structure is based on the presence of a heterocycle, a sulfur atom and an aromatic ring supporting a strong acidic group, which is negatively charged on all range of working pH. The ligand is called mercaptobenzimidazole sulfonic acid. Once attached chemically on a solid matrix, it adsorbs antibodies in physiological ionic strength at a pH between 5 and 5.5. Elution takes place when raising the pH to 8.5-9.5.

The mechanism of action is as complex as the one described for mercaptoethyl pyridine, although the adsorption does not happen by hydrophobic association. The sulfur atom and the heterocycle are both important for the selective adsorption of antibodies, while the presence of a sulfonate group, which is negatively charged during the adsorption phase (pH 5.0 – 5.5) contributes for the repulsion of albumin and other molecular species. IgG are therefore selectively separated in a single step at a purity above 85-90 % starting from whole undiluted serum. Traces of transferrin are among small impurities found in the IgG fraction. Figure 4.3 shows the separation of rat monoclonal IgG from a crude whole supernatant from a hybridoma cell culture in the presence of 10% fetal bovine serum.

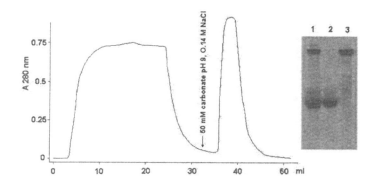

Figure 4.3. Separation of rat monoclonal antibodies from hybridoma cell culture supernatant in the presence of 10% fetal bovine serum using MBI HyperCel. Loading was performed after lowering the pH of the sample to 5.2. Elution of antibodies was accomplished by raising the pH to 9 with a 50 mM carbonate buffer containing 140 mM sodium chloride. Insert represents SDS electrophoresis analysis of crude supernatant (1), flowthrough (2) and eluted IgG fraction (3). The purified antibodies show trace impurities of transferrin; no albumin adsorption occurred.

Taken together mercaptoethyl pyridine and mercaptobenzimidazole sulfonic acids are complementary ligands for the purification of antibodies as demonstrated in the case of milk whey (results not shown). They can be advantageously used in direct tandem mode with no change in pH between columns.

4. ELECTRON DONOR-ACCEPTOR INTERACTION

The formation of neutral molecular complexes under the influence of weak attractive forces is at the basis of a large number of mechanisms of protein adsorption on solid phases. This interaction is generated from the electron donor-acceptor properties of the interacting moieties: the immobilized ligand and the protein to separate. It is on this principle that some aromatic compounds in aqueous solution interact with each other. Although in this case forces involved are of hydrophobic nature, other forces like electron donor-acceptor complexes contribute to the attraction of partners.

First observations indicate that such interaction would involve aromatic or heterocyclic compounds; however, it is not necessary that the ligand contain aromatic ring systems.

Ligands containing sulfur and nitrogen can easily act as interacting centers for amino acid residues at the surface of proteins.

In the case of antibody separation, thiophilic ligands and immobilized metal ions have characteristics that are close to the formation of complexes depending on the exchange of electrons between specific sites. They are both considered in the following lines as interesting means for the separation of antibodies.

4.1   Thiophilic ligands for antibody adsorption

The interest of sulfur atoms for ligand adsorption chromatography was recognized several decades ago [Porath, 1960; Gelotte, 1960]. The presence of one or several sulfur atoms on given ligands compared to the same with oxygen atoms instead, gave the first indications that the sulphur atoms have an effect on the adsorption of proteins. The strength of this interaction appeared dependent on the electrophilic and nucleophilic substituents of the ligand, supporting thus the hypothesis that electron donor-acceptor complexes were responsible for the interaction. In this context it was found that resins carrying vinylsulfone groups reacted with 2-mercaptoethanol (two sulphur atoms in the ligand structure) were good adsorbents for antibodies [Porath, 1985; Hutchens, 1986; Porath, 1987].

Elution patterns of whole human serum on this type of solid phase media in the presence of high concentrations of ammonium sulfate evidenced selective protein desorption. Good separation was observed for immunoglobulins G from both α1-antitrypsin and α2-macroglobulin [Hutchens, 1986].

A large number of applications in the separation of antibodies by thiophilic chromatography have been described in the last decade. Konecny et al., 1994, described the separation of immunoglobulins G from bovine milk whey; other publications reported the separation of antibodies from cell culture supernatants [Birkenmeyer, 1992; Arguelles, 1999], from chicken eggs [Hanach, 1998] and from ascites fluid [Bog-Hansen, 1997].

Thiophilic chromatography has also been used for the separation of antibody subclasses [Bridonneau, 1993]

Thiophilic interaction with respect to antibody separation has also been investigated in more complex situations where the group vicinal to the thioether bond was a pyridine ring. It was observed that IgGs were adsorbed much strongly than when a phenyl group is present [Oscarson, 1990]; however, albumin was also part of adsorbed proteins. This investigation suggested that the more electron donor acceptors groups are present, the higher the affinity and the binding capacity for antibodies.

With this in mind the use of heterocyclic compounds for the synthesis of thiophilic ligands was further investigated [Porath, 1998]. It was demonstrated that heterocyclic compounds, attached to a solid matrix *via* a thioether bond, were able to adsorb some classes of proteins from serum, such as antibodies and α2-macroglobulin, but not albumin.

More recently, other heterocyclic compounds attached *via* divinylsulfone activation have been described as ligands for the purification of antibodies [Scholz, 1998a; Scholz, 1998b]. These derivatives allowed adsorbing antibodies without addition of lyotropic salts; desorption was accomplished by increasing the pH.

4.2 Immobilized metal affinity chromatography

Immobilized Metal Affinity Chromatography (IMAC) is based on the metal ion mediated interaction with proteins. To achieve this interaction on solid phase, metal ions are adsorbed on a chelating resin and the resulting solid phase used for protein adsorption. Chelation of metal ions occurs *via* the intervention of selected ligands chemically attached on the matrix. The most popular chelating ligand is iminodiacetic acid. For more details on these affinity mediated resins see Table 4.3 [Chaga, 2001 and Gaberc-Porekar, 2001 for reviews].

Table 4.3: Common chelating molecules for metal ion immobilization

Chelating ligand	Coordination	Metal ions
Iminodiacetic acid	Tridentate	Cu^{++}, Zn^{++}, Ni^{++}, Co^{++}
Notrilotriacetic acid	Tetradentate	Ni^{++}
Carboxymethyl aspartic acid	Tetradentate	Ca^{++}, Co^{++}
Aminohydroxamic acid	Bidentate	Fe^{+++}
Salicylaldehyde	Bidentate	Cu^{++}
N-(2-pyridylmethyl)amino acetate	Tridentate	Cu^{++}
Ortho-phosphoserine	Tridentate	Fe^{+++}, Al^{+++}

In immobilized metal affinity chromatography protein adsorption is dependent on the coordination between a transition metal ions and an electron donor group of the protein.

Common transition metals that have electron-pair acceptors are Cu^{++}, Co^{++}, Ni^{++}, Zn^{++}, Fe^{+++}. These metal ions are strongly adsorbed on chelating resins having electron donor atoms such as N, S, and O. Remaining coordination sites on the chelated metal ions are occupied by molecules of water and can be exchanged with electron-donor groups of the protein residues. The primary protein residue to interact with transition metal ions is histidine; however other aminoacids such as, Arg, Asp, Cys, Glu, Met and Tyr can participate for protein retention on the solid phase media.

Other groups such as Phe, Trp and Tyr appear to contribute as well when they are close to a histidyl residue. Conditions of interactions are when the histidyl group is protonated, in other word when the pH is neutral or slightly alkaline.

As a result of the presence in their structure of a highly conserved histidyl cluster at the junctures of CH2 and CH3 domains of Fc fragment [Burton, 1985], antibodies interact quite strongly and specifically with these resins. Therefore they are easily adsorbed and separated from a variety of feedstocks [Porath, 1983; Sharma, 1997].

Separation of antibody by metal chelate affinity chromatography is influenced by several parameters such as the nature of immobilized chelating group, the immobilized metal ion, and the pH environment.

El Rassi and Horváth, 1986, explained the retention of proteins on metal-chelate sorbents as influenced by several parameters that are connected with the transition metal ion, the presence of salt in the mobile phase and an electrostatic influence.

Antibody interaction generally occurs with nickel ions [Sulkowsky, 1985] or copper ions [Li-Chan, 1990] as well as cobalt ions. Polyclonal IgGs were efficiently recovered from low concentration cheese whey at high binding capacity and purity. IgG was found to be able to competitively displace less tightly bound proteins such as β-lactoglobulin, α-lactalbumin, serum albumin and lactoperoxidase, during whey loading.

A typical example is the purification of humanized monoclonal antibodies [Sulkowsky, 1985]: after filtration of feed stock, IgG was adsorbed directly and eluted by a descending pH gradient from 7.5 to 4.25. Purity obtained was about 90%; reported recovery was greater than 90%.

As a general rule adsorption of antibodies on metal chelating resins occurs best in slightly alkaline pHs, which selectively favour the adsorption of antibodies. This step may be performed in the presence of 0.5-1 M sodium chloride that prevents weak adsorption of other proteins [Hale, 1994].

Several options are available for the elution of antibodies. Among them is the decrease of the buffer pH to 3.8-4.5, and the addition of competitive molecules such as imidazol, histidine or histidine analogs. Other effective chemicals capable of desorbing antibodies are chelating agents such as EDTA, EGTA and iminodiacetic acid. They act as very effective sequestering agents to remove the metal ions and consequently they desorb antibodies. These latter are, however, contaminated by metal ions. Known contaminants of purified antibodies using metal chelate affinity chromatography include traces of transferrin and albumin.

5.   METHOD DEVELOPMENT FOR THE DESIGN OF A SEPARATION PROCESS

Production of antibodies using available expression tools (cells, transgenic animals, transgenic plants) requires numerous trials of cloning and expression to generate suitable antibody with appropriate biological specificity and affinity. Most generally, expression of a novel antibody is performed at very small scale and the level of expression is frequently low at this stage. Therefore the number of samples generated for antibody separation is high while the amount of available material for separation trials is very limited.

In this respect it is difficult to figure out how to purify the expressed antibody from crude feedstock using liquid column chromatography. Common approaches for process development are to prepare different columns and then to run separations under multiple conditions. In this manner, it is possible to identify the appropriate parameters allowing capture of the antibody while leaving in the flow-through the maximum number of impurities. Determination of the purity of each chromatographic fraction or collected peak is then performed by classical electrophoresis methods or by analytical HPLC. This process is particularly time consuming and requires large volumes of crude feedstocks.

In order to rapidly reach optimized conditions of separation, heuristics have been suggested [Ostlund, 1986; Bonnerjea, 1986; Wheelwright, 1989]. However, they rarely consider composition of biological fluids, which is very critical since such fluids are very complex and variable, and as such, not subject to discretionary changes.

Another approach in designing a process is to make separation mapping. This is best accomplished when employing automated chromatographs that make use of sophisticated software capable of elucidating ideal separation conditions from complex matrix combining different parameters [Lewis, 1992; Patapoff, 1993]. Nevertheless, the selection of optimized separation condition is ultimately judged by an accurate electrophoresis analysis or HPLC data of collected fractions.

Usually a process is decomposed in three main steps called initial capture, fractionation and final polishing. The capture of the antibody by biospecific interaction is an operation that does not generally require a great deal of effort for the definition of conditions. This is the case for instance of protein A resins. However, after this selective capture phase the separation of remaining impurities is always challenging. An example of capture-fractionation-polishing is given on Figure 4.1.

Recently, developments have been made in attempting to use functionalized surfaces associated with mass spectroscopy strategies towards the development of process chromatography protocols [Weinberger, 2002; Shiloach, 2003]. This method has been shown to be effective, facile, and rapid for the separation of antibody fragments and other proteins. The volume of sample is minimal (in the range of µlitres) while clearly predicting optimal separation conditions directly implementable to chromatographic columns. These functionalized arrays are called "protein biochips", and the adsorption-desorption of extremely small amounts of proteins can be evaluated directly by mass spectrometry.

Briefly the process consists in a deposition of a protein mixture upon an array's functionalized surface, an interaction occurs between the array's surface and proteins, resulting in adsorption of certain species. The application of gradient wash conditions to the surface of these arrays produces a step-wise elution of retained compounds akin to that accomplished while utilizing columns for liquid chromatography separations. Retained proteins on the surface are then analyzed by mass spectrometry directly from the chromatographic surface.

Several studies demonstrated that protein biochips can be used to identify conditions of pH and ionic strength that support selective retention/elution of target proteins and impurity components from ion exchange as well as IMAC and hydrophobic surfaces. Such conditions give corresponding behaviour when using chromatographic sorbents under elution chromatography conditions (Figure 4.4).

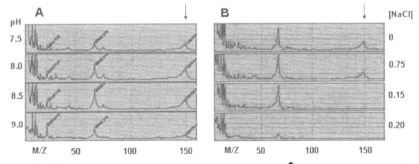

Figure 4.4. Mass spectrometry results using ProteinChip® Array technology for the determination of separation conditions of a mouse IgG1 monoclonal antibody from a cell culture supernatant. Chromatographic surface supported quaternary amine groups. pH 8 was selected from a first pH screening study (A). At pH 8 different ionic strength conditions were tried (B) to obtain optimal loading conditions and desorption conditions: 0.15 M sodium chloride was selected (no presence of IgG but albumin was still adsorbed). Arrows indicate the positioning of IgG.

The methods involving chip chromatographic surfaces along with mass spectrometry analysis of retained proteins can therefore be used to predict conditions for regular chromatography. This method was applied to the separation of a Fab antibody fragment expressed in *Escherichia coli* [Weinberger, 2002] as well as to the separation of recombinant endostatin as expressed in supernatant of *Pichia pastoris* cultures [Shiloach, 2003]. This separation process design combined with mass spectrometry not only provides the definition of separation conditions, but also brings information of purity of the adsorbed molecules (identifiable by its molecular mass) avoiding thus the use of electrophoresis analysis.

This approach can easily be utilized for devising the separation process of antibodies starting from very small volumes of crude feedstock. The first step is to select the protein chip array appropriate for the separation of the antibody. Once the chip surface is selected, the following operation consists of finding the best conditions of pH capable to discriminate between the target antibody and protein impurities. A second step will give data on the impact of ionic strength variations at the selected pH on conditions of adsorption and desorption that can be easily transferred to liquid column chromatography.

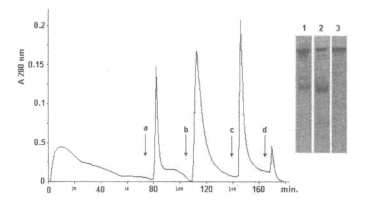

Figure 4.5. Separation of murine monoclonal immunoglobulin G1 from a cell culture supernatant containing albumin, transferrin and insulin on a Q HyperZ column. Selection of sorbent and of separation conditions of pH and of ionic strength were from predictive study on ProteinChip® Arrays (see Figure 4). Elution of proteins was accomplished by discrete increase of sodium chloride in a 50 mM Tris-HCl buffer, pH 8. "a" to "d" arrows indicate elution steps at respectively 75, 150, 200 and 400 mM sodium chloride. Insert represents SDS electrophoresis analysis of mixtures of IgG, albumin and insulin (1), crude cell culture supernatant (2) and eluted fraction at 75 mM sodium chloride (3).

Figure 4.5 illustrates an example of process development for the separation of antibodies from a cell culture supernatant.

When the starting material is as complex as a serum with thousand of proteins, a pre-fractionation may be preferred before the definition of separation conditions.

6.   CONCLUSION AND FUTURE PROSPECTS

For a number of years, disappointing therapeutic results prevented the commercial development of antibodies. On the contrary antibodies used in diagnostics developed extensively in diversity and applications. In spite of diminished enthusiasm in the therapeutically usable antibodies, more and more performant methodologies have been developed involving innovative approaches in the design of sorbents for chromatography.

More recently, with the demonstration of spectacular results in therapy with humanized antibodies under their different forms, the separation activity around antibody production grew spectacularly.

With the advent of an exponential growth in antibody-based applications, new production methods are under accelerated development. Fermentation capabilities have increased significantly, expression levels of cultured cells are improved and other production methods involving transgenic animals and plants are under investigation to increase the productivity.

In this situation, extraction, separation and purification of antibodies will undoubtedly follow and evolve in parallel with the evolution of applications and of market needs.

The design of an antibody purification process will consider, more than today, the final utilization of the molecule. For example, the degree of purity will not be the same if the antibody is to be used for research purposes, for diagnostic or for long term therapeutic applications.

The process design should also consider the scale of the final process in order to meet economical requirements.

When using chromatography, one of the major points to consider is related to the use of water. Liquid chromatography actually involves large volumes of aqueous buffers and a way to save part of them is to adjust conditions between columns so as to use similar buffers and to decrease the column volumes. Water savings can also be achieved by other different ways. Absence of dilution of original feedstocks is one direct possibility to save water consumption. However, to comply with this statement chromatography sorbents must be compatible with physiological ionic strength for antibody adsorption. This is the case with the use of affinity or pseudo-affinity capturing sorbents. Ion exchange would then be used as a second separation step. Saving water consumptions can also be achieved by choosing high binding capacity and easily cleanable resins.

Finally, since specific impurities are to be eliminated for regulatory reasons, the process design configuration must be part of a global approach. Compatibility from one column to another, thus eliminating the necessity to dialyze or to dilute, is an important source of economy as well.

Specificity will more and more be a target to diminish the volumes of the columns required and consequent volumes of buffers. The last column, which is intended for polishing, should adsorb impurities instead of the antibody. In such a configuration the volume of the column will also be reduced in size.

Another observed trend is the direct capture of antibodies from the crude feedstock in the presence of cells or cell debris. Feedstocks will come continuously directly from fermentors without the need of cell separation. In this configuration virtual filters may be placed on the top of the fermentor, or cells are pushed to travel through the beads of a column used as a fluidized bed mode. In both cases the bead surface is modified in such a way so that antibodies are adsorbed very specifically in physiological conditions but cells are not.

Technologies converge unavoidably towards the design of sorbents with characteristics that are already defined. Selectivity is to be as good as biospecific interactions, binding capacity must be as high as ion exchangers, cleanability has to be absolute with strong caustic agents, leakage must not occur and cost of column must be as low as possible. In this context it is anticipated that the design of chromatographic material will continue to make progress.

ACKNOWLEDGEMENTS

The author wishes to thank Dr Lee Lomas (Ciphergen Biosystems Inc, Fremont, CA) for his critical review of the manuscript and to Dr Luc Bourgeois and Pierre Girot (all from Ciphergen-Biosepra, Cergy, France) for providing technical data.

REFERENCES

Akerstrom B., Bjorck L. A physicochemical study of protein G, a molecule with unique immunoglobulin G-binding properties. J. Biol. Chem. 1986; 261: 10240-7.

Arguelles M.E., Alonso M., Garcia-Suarez M.D., Barneo L., Sampedro A., de los Toyos J.R. Performance of thiophilic adsorption chromatography in the purification of rat IgG2b monoclonal antibodies from serum- and protein-free culture supernatants. Biomed. Chromatogr. 1999; 13: 379-81.

Bazin H., Xhurdebise L. M., Burtonboy G., Lebacq A. M., De Clercq L., Cormont F. Rat monoclonal antibodies. I. Rapid purification from in vitro culture supernatants. J. Immunol. Methods. 1984a; 66: 261-9.

Bazin H., Cormont F., De Clercq L. Rat monoclonal antibodies. II. A rapid and efficient method of purification from ascitic fluid or serum. J. Immunol. Methods. 1984b; 71: 9-16.

Belew M., Juntti N., Larsson A., Porath J. A one-step purification method for monoclonal antibodies based on salt-promoted adsorption chromatography on a 'thiophilic' adsorbent., J. Immunol. Meth. 1987; 102: 173-82.

Birkenmeier S.B., Kopperschlager G. Application of phase partitioning and thiophilic adsorption chromatography to the purification of monoclonal antibodies from cell culture fluid. J. Immunol. Meth. 1992; 149: 165-61.

Bog-Hansen T.C. Separation of monoclonal antibodies from cell culture supernatants and ascites fluid using thiophilic agarose. Mol. Biotechnol. 1997; 8: 279-81.

Bonnerjea J., Oh S., Hoare M., Dunnill P., Protein purification: the right step at the right time. Biotechnology. 1986; 4: 954-58.

Boschetti E., Jungbauer A. "Separation of antibodies by liquid chromatography." In: *Handbook of Biosepartions* Vol 2, S. Ahuja ed. Acad. Press, 2000, pp 535-632.

Boschetti, E. The use of thiophilic chromatography for antibody purification: a review. J. Biochem. Biophys. Meth. 2001a; 49: 361-89.

Boschetti E., Guerrier L. Purification of antibodies by HCIC and impact of ligand structure. I. J. BioChromatogr. 2001b; 6: 269-83.

Boschetti E., Girot P. "Ion exchange interaction biochromatography." In: *Biochromatography, Theory and Practice.* M.A. Vijiayalakshmi ed. Taylor and Francis publisher., 2002a, pp. 24-45.

Boschetti E. Separation of antibodies by hydrophobic charge induction chromatography. Trends Biotechnol. 2002b; 20: 333-7.

Bridonneau P., Lederer F. Bahaviour of immunoglobulin G subclasses on thiophilic gels: comparison with hydrophobic interaction chromatography. J. Chromatogr. 1993; 616: 197-204.

Burton D. R. Immunoglobulins G: functional sites. Mol. Immunol. 1985; 22: 161-206.

Carlsson M., Hedin A., Inganas M., Harfast B., Blomberg, F. Purification of in vitro produced mouse monoclonal antibodies. A two- step procedure utilizing cation exchange chromatography and gel filtration. J. Immunol. Methods. 1985; 79: 89-98.

Carlson J., Janson J. C., Sparrman M. « Affinity Chromatography." In: *Protein purification: principles, high resolution methods, and applications.* A John Wiley & sons, Inc., New York. 1988.

Chaga G.S. Twenty-five years of immobilized metal ion affinity chromatography: past present and future. J. Biochem. Biophys. Meth. 2001; 49: 313-34.

Chen F. M., Naeve G. S., Epstein A. L. Comparison of mono Q, superose-6, and ABx fast protein liquid chromatography for the purification of IgM monoclonal antibodies. J. Chromatogr. 1988; 444: 153-64.

Danielsson A., Ljunglof A., Lindblom H. One-step purification of monoclonal IgG antibodies from mouse ascites. An evaluation of different adsorption techniques using high performance liquid chromatography. J. Immunol. Methods. 1988; 115: 79-88.

Duffy S., Moellering B. J., Prior G. M., Doyle K. R., Prior C. P. Recovery of Therapeutic-grade of antibodies: Protein A and ion exchange chromatography. BioPharm. 1989; June: 35-47.

Ey P. L., Prowse S. J., Jenkin C. R. Isolation of pure IgG1, IgG2a and IgG2b immunoglobulins from mouse serum using protein A-sepharose. Immunochemistry. 1978; 15: 429-36.

El-Kak A., Manjiny S. Vijayalakshmi M. A. Interaction of immunoglobulin G(IgG) with immobilized histidine: Mechanistic and kinetic aspects. J. Chromatogr. 1992; 604: 29-37.

El-Rassi Z., Horvath, C. Metal chelate-interaction chromatography of proteins with iminodiacetic acid-bonded stationary phases on silica support. J. Chromatogr. 1986; 359: 241-53.

Fuglistaller P. Comparison of immunoglobulin binding capacities and ligand leakage using eight different protein A affinity chromatography matrices. J. Immunol. Methods. 1989; 124: 171-7.

Fassina G., Verdoliva A., Palombo G., Ruvo M. Cassani G. Immunoglobulin specificity of TG19318: a novel synthetic ligand for antibody affinity purification. J. Mol. Recognit. 1998; 11: 128-33.

Fassina G, Ruvo M, Palombo G, Verdoliva A, Marino M. Novel ligands for the affinity-chromatographic purification of antibodies. J. Biochem. Biophys. Methods. 2001;49:481-90.

Gaberc-Porekar V., Menart V. Perspectives of immobilized-metal affinity chromatography. J. Biochem. Biophys. Meth. 2001; 49: 335-60.

Gelotte B. Studies on gel filtration sorption properties of the bed material Sephadex. J. Chromatogr. 1960; 3: 330-42.

Godfrey M.A., Kwasowwski P., Clift R., Marks V. Assessment of the suitability of commercially available SpA affinity solid phases for the purification of murine monoclonal antibodies at process scale. J. Immunol. Meth. 1993; 160: 97-105.

Guerrier L., Flayeux I., Schwarz A., Fassina G., Boschetti, E. IRIS 97: an innovating Protein A-peptidomimetic solid phase media for antibody purification. J. Mol. Recognit. 1998; 11: 1-3.

Hale J. E., Beidler D. E. Purification of humanized murine and murine monoclonal antibodies using immobilized metal-affinity chromatography. Anal. Biochem. 1994; 222: 29-33.

Hansen P., Scoble J.A., Hanson B., Hoogenraad N.J. Isolation and purification of immunoglobulins from chicken eggs using thiophilic interaction chromatography. J. Immunol. Meth. 1998; 215: 1-7.

Hutchens T.W., Porath J. Thiophilic adsorption of immunoglobulins - analysis of conditions optimal for selective immobilization and purification. Anal. Biochem. 1986; 159: 217-26.

Jiskoot W, Van Hertrooij JJ, Klein Gebbinck JW, Van der Velden-de Groot T, Crommelin DJ, Beuvery EC. Two-step purification of a murine monoclonal antibody intended for therapeutic application in man. Optimisation of purification conditions and scaling up. J. Immunol. Methods. 1989;124:143-56.

Konecny P., Brown R.J., Scouten W.H. Chromatographic purification of immunoglobulin G from bovine milk whey. J. Chromatogr. 1994;673: 45-53.

Lewis J.A., Lommen D.C., Raddatz W.D., Dolan J.W., Snyder L.R., Molnar I.J. Computer simulation for the prediction of separation as a function of pH for reversed-phase high-performance liquid chromatography. I. Accuracy of a theory-based model. J. Chromatogr. 1992; 502: 183-95.

Li R., Dowd V., Stewart D. J., Burton S. J., and Lowe C. R. Design, synthesis and application of a Protein A mimetic. Nat. Biotechnol. 1998; 16: 190-5.

Li-Chan E., Kwan L., Nakai S. Isolation of immunoglobulins by competitive displacement of cheese whey proteins during metal chelate interaction chromatography. J. Diary Sci. 1990; 73: 2075-86.

Lihme A., Bendix-Hansen M. Protein A mimetic for large scale monoclonal antibody purification. Biotechnology Laboratory 1997;15: 30-1.

McLaren R. D., Prosser C. G., Grieve R. C., Borissenko M. The use of caprylic acid for the extraction of the immunoglobulin fraction from egg yolk of chickens immunised with ovine alpha-lactalbumin. J. Immunol. Methods. 1994; 177: 175-84.

Mohan S. B., Lyddiatt A. "Recent developments in affinity separation technologies." In *Affinity separations.* IRL Press, Oxford. 1997; pp1-38.

Moks T., Abrahmsen L., Nilsson B., Hellman U., Sjoquist J., Uhlen M. Staphylococcal protein A consists of five IgG-binding domains. Eur. J Biochem. 1986; 156: 637-43.

Necina R., Amatschek K., Jungbauer A. Capture of human monoclonal antibodies from cell culture supernatant by ion exchange media exhibiting high charge density. Biotechnol. Bioeng. 1998; 60: 679-98.

Ngo T. T., Khatter N., and Avid A. L. A synthetic ligand affinity gel mimicking immobilized bacterial antibody receptor for purification of immunoglobulin G. J. Chromatogr. 1992; 597: 101-9.

Ngo T.T. Rapid purification of immunoglobulin G using aza-arenophilic chromatography: novel mode of protein solid phase interactions. J. Chromatogr. 1994; 662: 351-6.

Nilson B. H., Logdberg L., Kastern W., Bjorck L., Akerstrom B. Purification of antibodies using protein L-binding framework structures in the light chain variable domain. J. Immunol. Meth. 1993; 164: 33-40.

Oscarson S., Porath J. Protein Chromatography with pyridine- and alkyl- thioether-based agarose adsorbents. J. Chromatogr. 1990; 499: 235-47.

Ostlund C. Large-scale purification of monoclonal antibodies. Trends in Biotechnology. 1986; 4: 288-293.

Palombo G., Verdoliva A., Fassina G. Affinity purification of immunoglobulin M using a novel synthetic ligand. J. Chromatogr. 1998; 715: 137-45.

Patapoff T.W., Marnsy R.J., Lee W.A. The application of size exclusion chromatography and computer simulation to study the thermodynamic and kinetic parameters for short-lived dissociable protein aggregates. Anal. Biochem. 1993 ; 212 : 71-8 .

Peng L., Calton G. J., Burnett J. W. Stability of antibody attachement in immunosorbent chromatography. Enzyme Microbiol. Technol.. 1986; 8: 681-5.

Porath J., Biochem Biophys Acta, 1960; 50: 193.

Porath J., Olin B. Immobilized metal ion affinity adsorption and immobilized metal ion affinity chromatography of biomaterials. Serum protein affinities for gel immobilized iron and nickel ions. Biochemistry. 1983; 22: 1621-30.

Porath J., Maisano F., Belew M. Thiophilic adsorption - a new method for protein fractionation. FEBS Lett. 1985;185: 306-10.

Porath J., Belew M. 'Thiophilic' interaction and the selective adsorption of proteins. Tibtech. 1987; 5: 225-9.

Porath J., Oscarsson S. A new kind of "thiophilic" electron-donor-acceptor adsorbent., Makromol. Chem. Macromol. Synth. 1988; 17: 359-71.

Scholz G. H., Wippich P., Leistner S., Huse K. Salt-independent binding of antibodies from human serum to thiophilic heterocyclic ligands. J. Chromatogr. 1998a; 709: 189-96.

Scholz G. H., Vieweg S., Leistner S., J., S., Scherbaum W. A., Huse K. A simplified procedure for the isolation of immunoglobulins from human serum using a novel type of thiophilic gel at low salt concentration. J. Immunol. Meth. 1998b; 219: 109-18.

Sharma S. K. "Designer affinity purification of recombinant proteins." In: *Affinity separations, a practical approach.* Oxford University Press, Oxford. 1997, pp197-218.

Shiloach J., Santambien P., Trinh L., Schapman A., Boschetti E. Endostatin capture from *P. pastoris* culture on fluidized bed: from on-chip process optimization to application. J. Chromatogr. 2003; 790: 327-36.

Sulkowsky E. Purification of proteins by IMAC. Trends Biotechnol. 1985; 3: 1-3.

Teng SF, Sproule K, Hussain A, Lowe CR. A strategy for the generation of biomimetic ligands for affinity chromatography. Combinatorial synthesis and biological evaluation of an IgG binding ligand. J. Mol. Recognit. 1999;12:67-75.

Teng SF, Sproule K, Husain A, Lowe CR. Affinity chromatography on immobilized "biomimetic" ligands. Synthesis, immobilization and chromatographic assessment of an immunoglobulin G-binding ligand. J. Chromatogr. 2000; 740:1-15.

Weinberger S., Boschetti E., Santambien P., Brenac V. Surface enhanced laser desorption / ionization retentate chromatography mass spectrometry (SELDI-RC-MS): a new method for rapid development of process chromatography conditions. J. Chromatogr. 2002; 782: 307-16.

Wheelwright S.M. The design of downstream process for large-scale protein purification. J. Biotechnology. 1989; 11: 89-102.

Chapter 5

NOVEL HIV NEUTRALIZING ANTIBODIES SELECTED FROM PHAGE DISPLAY LIBRARIES

Maxime Moulard[*], Mei-Yun Zhang[#,%] and Dimiter S. Dimitrov[#]

[*]BioCytex, 140 Chemin de l'Armée d'Afrique, 13010 Marseille, France; [#]Laboratory of Experimental and Computational Biology, Center for Cancer Research, NCI-Frederick, NIH, Bldg 469, Rm 246, P.O. Box B, Miller Drive, Frederick, MD 21702-1201, USA; [%]BRP, SAIC-Frederick, Inc., Bldg 469, Rm 131, P.O. Box B, Miller Drive, Frederick, MD 21702-1201, USA

1.   INTRODUCTION

Neutralizing antibodies play a major role in host defense against viral infections. Passive administration of antibodies specific for HIV-1 can protect monkeys from infections mediated by the HIV-1 envelope glycoprotein (Env) in a concentration dependent manner (Shibata et al., 1999; Baba et al., 2000; Ruprecht et al., 2001; Xu et al., 2002; Veazey et al., 2003; Burton, 2002; Ferrantelli and Ruprecht, 2002; Mascola et al., 1999; Mascola et al., 2000; Mascola, 2002; Parren et al., 2001). In some of these experiments human monoclonal antibodies (hmAbs) were used that exhibit potent and broad HIV neutralizing activity in vitro (Burton, 1997; Burton, 2002; Ferrantelli and Ruprecht, 2002). Recent clinical trials found that two of these broadly HIV neutralizing hmAbs (nhmAbs), 2F5 and 2G12, could produce a modest decrease in viral load without side effects in humans (Armbruster et al., 2002; Stiegler et al., 2002). However, the potency of 2F5 and 2G12 used in combination in this clinical trial was not sufficient to reduce the HIV-1 plasma RNA levels to the low levels observed after treatment with HAART (Stiegler et al., 2002). Increases in the potency of the currently available broadly HIV nhmAbs and the development of new neutralizing hmAbs might be helpful here although problems associated with neutralization escape are likely to be severe in any attempts to use antibodies therapeutically. Importantly, finding immunogens that are able to elicit broadly HIV nhmAbs could be facilitated by the exploration of the interaction of these antibodies with the Env - an approach known as "retrovaccinology" (Burton, 2002). However, only a few broadly cross-reactive HIV nhmAbs have been identified to date and efforts to use mimetics of their epitopes or portions of the epitopes as immunogens are ongoing but of limited success so far (Zwick et al., 2001a). The identification of new broadly cross-reactive HIV nhmAbs and their conserved epitopes is therefore of obvious importance for the development of effective HIV vaccines.

HIV specific polyclonal antibodies can be isolated from the serum of humans infected with HIV or immunized with HIV antigens, and monoclonal antibodies can be produced by hybridomas or identified by screening of phage display libraries (Parren and Burton, 1997). During the last decade the development and screening of libraries from displayed Fabs or scFvs linked to their genotype has become a major methodology for identification of high affinity hmAbs. One of the most potent and well characterized broadly HIV nhmAbs, IgG1 b12, that recognizes the gp120 subunit of the Env was identified by screening of a human antibody phage display library and shown to neutralize a variety of primary HIV-1 isolates (Burton et al., 1994). Recently, another broadly cross-reactive HIV nhmAb, Z13, that recognizes the gp41 subunit of the Env, was also identified by screening of an antibody phage display library (Zwick et al., 2001b). Only three other potent broadly HIV nhmAbs, 2G12, 2F5 and 4E10, have been described until recently. Here, we review our recent work on identification and characterization of new HIV-1 nhmAbs selected from phage display libraries that could contribute to the development of new treatments and vaccines against HIV.

2.   PHAGE DISPLAY METHODOLOGY

Antibody fragments, as Fabs or single chain Fv (scFv), have been among the first proteins to be displayed on the surface of a filamentous bacteriophage (McCafferty et al., 1990). In antibody phage display, antibody V-gene repertoires are batch-cloned into the phage genome as a fusion to the gene encoding one of the phage coat proteins (pIII, pVI or pVIII). Upon expression, the coat protein fusion is incorporated into new phage particles that are assembled in the periplasmic space of infected bacteria. Expression of the fusion product and its subsequent incorporation into the mature phage coat results in the surface-displayed recombinant antibodies, while its genetic material resides within the phage particle. The connection between antibody genotype and phenotype allows the enrichment of phage particles specific for a given antigen using selection based on antigen-antibody interactions. The success of any specific antibody isolation depends largely on the antibody gene repertoire complexity, antibody display methodology, selection procedure (biopanning) and characterization of specific antibody clones (screening).

2.1 Phage display libraries

Antibody libraries can be produced either from antibody V-gene repertoires derived from human or animal donors or from synthetic or semi-synthetic antibody V-gene repertoires constructed in vitro. Libraries made from immunized animals (immune libraries) compared to libraries (naïve libraries) obtained from antigen-naive animals are biased toward antibody genes encoding antibodies recognizing the target antigens (Marks et al., 1991; Williamson et al., 1993b). Thus specific antibodies can be selected using a relatively small, random combinatorial V-gene library derived from an immunized donor (Clackson et al., 1991; Burton et al., 1991). 'Naïve' libraries should have larger diversity ($>10^{10}$ clones) to isolate antibodies with affinity similar to those selected from relatively small libraries made from immunized donors. Antibodies from 'naïve' repertoires can be produced against self-antigens and have relatively fast off-rates (Griffiths et al., 1993) that may require affinity maturation for improvement of binding (Schier et al., 1996c; Schier et al., 1996a; Schier et al., 1996b; Schier and Marks, 1996). Antibodies to several antigens can also be selected from immune libraries, e.g., a single combinatorial library from an HIV-1 infected patient who had been exposed to other viruses was successfully used to generate human Fabs against a plethora of viruses including HIV-1, CMV, HSV-1, HSV-2, RSV, Rubella and varicella zoster (Williamson et al., 1993a). Human monoclonal Fabs to viral antigens have also been selected from combinatorial IgA libraries (Moreno et al., 1995) and IgM libraries (Toran et al., 1999).

The first Fab phage display library used for selection of anti-HIV hmAbs was prepared from the bone marrow of a 31-year-old homosexual HIV-1-infected male who had been asymptomatic for 6 years (Burton et al., 1991). One of the most potent and broadly HIV neutralizing hmAb Fab, b12, was selected from this library and later converted to IgG1 that exhibited even higher neutralizing activity against primary isolates (Burton et al., 1994). Several other antibody libraries have been prepared from HIV-1-infected patients (Parren and Burton, 1997). An important consideration for selection of patients for preparation of antibody libraries is the existence of high titer of potent and broadly HIV neutralizing antibodies in their serum. Two libraries were prepared from HIV seropositive donors (FDA2 and DS) whose serum was able to neutralize both T-cell line adapted viruses (TCLA) and selection of primary isolates (PI) (Vujcic and Quinnan, Jr., 1995; Parren et al., 1998). The binding of IgG from both patients to Env expressed at the surface of chronically infected cells (Moulard et al., 2000) was strong (Fig 5.1). The binding of the FDA2 patient serum IgG was significantly higher than IgG prepared from a mixture of 25 patient immunoglobulins (HIVIg).

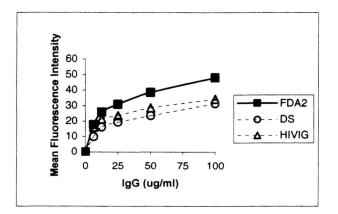

Figure 5.1. Binding capacity of immunoglobulin preparations to infected cells. T-cell line H9 was chronically infected with the TCLA X4 HIV-1$_{MN}$ isolate. Infected cells were immunolabeled with purified IgGs from FDA2, DS or from a pool of sera (HIVIg) at the indicated concentrations. The amount of bound antibodies was measured by flow cytometry and represented in arbitrary units of mean fluorescence intensity.

Purified immunoglobulins from FDA2 sera were also shown to bind to viral particles very efficiently in an assay described recently (Poignard et al., 2003). Purified immunoglobulins from FDA2 and HIVIg were used and compared to anti-HIV-1 hmAbs for binding to the virus (Fig.5.2). Mabs IgG1b12 (CD4-dependent), 2G12 (CD4-independent), and 17b (CD4-induced) were used as control. While the binding of the viral particle to IgG1b12 was inhibited by CD4 preincubation with the virus, the binding to 17b was enhanced by CD4 preincubation in the same experimental condition. As expected binding of the virus to the mAb 2G12 was unaffected. The amount of captured virus was more significantly increased with the FDA2 derived immunoglobulins than with the bulk from HIVIg. The results from the virus capture assay further argue for the presence of antibodies with high affinity for the HIV-1 gp120.

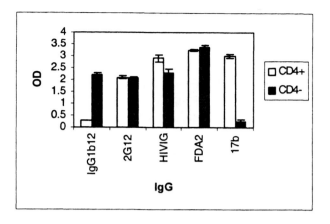

Figure 5.2. Virus capture assay. HIV-1$_{MN}$ was captured on ELISA plates coated with goat anti-human IgG Fc-specific Ab and anti-gp120 Abs or IgG from FDA2 or HIVIg serum. The quantity of p24 captured on the plate was measured as described in (Poignard et al., 2003).

Taken together, the data supported the hypothesis that FDA2 serum contains high concentration of antibodies that are able to bind efficiently Envs. A phage display library from FDA2 was prepared by conventional procedures (Barbas et al., 2001) and used for selection of X5 as described below. Another library was constructed using bone marrow obtained from three long term nonprogressors whose sera exhibited the broadest and most potent HIV-1 neutralization among 37 HIV-infected individuals (T. Evans et al., in preparation) and used for selection of m12,14,16,18 and 20 as summarized below.

2.2   Biopanning

An effective selection procedure is as important as antibody library construction for successful identification of high-affinity antibodies (Griffiths and Duncan, 1998). Selection of specific binders is usually performed by several cycles of incubation with the target antigen and amplification of the recombinant phage, a process referred as "biopanning". Biopanning allows phage to associate with the target antigen followed by extensive washing to remove non-specifically bound phage, then elution of the remaining particles, and reinfection of *E. coli* to monitor the recovery. Amplification of the eluted phage, followed by repetition of the selection process, allows enrichment of specific-binding clones (Barbas, III et al., 1991). Four to six rounds of panning are usually required to select phage of interest (Barbas et al., 2001).

Many different selection methods have been described, including biopanning on immobilized antigen coated onto solid supports such as ELISA plates, immunotubes or magnetic beads (solid-phase panning) (Clackson et al., 1991; Griffiths et al., 1994; Duenas et al., 1996; Marks et al., 1991; Sawyer et al., 1997), selection in solution using biotinylated antigen (solution-phase panning) (Hawkins et al., 1992), panning on fixed prokaryotic cells (Bradbury et al., 1993) or on mammalian cells (Cai and Garen, 1995) including cultured cells (Li et al., 2001) and primary cells (Ditzel et al., 2000; Williams et al., 2002), subtractive selection using sorting procedures, enrichment on tissue sections or pieces of tissue (de Kruif et al., 1995; Van Ewijk et al., 1997) and, in principle, selections using living animals (Trepel et al., 2002). Solid-phase panning and solution phase panning are commonly used if purified antigen is available. The choice of selection procedure depends on the properties of the targets and antibodies to be isolated. Panning against target antigen coated on magnetic beads is a useful approach for selection of antibodies specific for membrane glycoproteins (Sawyer et al., 1997). Strategies including epitope masking or specific blocking were shown to improve the selection process (Ditzel, 2002; Ditzel et al., 1995; Messmer and Thaler, 2001). An automated screening procedure has also been described recently (Hallborn and Carlsson, 2002).

In most cases one antigen is used in all rounds. Many viruses, including HIV, undergo rapid mutations as one of the strategies to escape host immune surveillance. To select for broadly cross-reactive antibodies recognizing conserved epitopes we hypothesized that selection of high-affinity antibodies against such epitopes can be facilitated by sequentially changing the antigen during the panning of phage display libraries and developed a methodology termed sequential antigen panning (SAP) (Zhang and Dimitrov, 2002, in preparation). This methodology was used for selection of new broadly HIV reactive hmAbs, m6,9,12,14,16,18 and 20, as described below.

3.   NEW HIV NEUTRALIZING HUMAN MONOCLONAL ANTIBODIES

3.1   Antibodies Selected by Soluble Recombinant Monomeric gp120ΔV3$_{JRFL}$

Recombinant gp120ΔV3 from HIV-1$_{JRFL}$, a gp120 which has been deleted for the V3-loop, was selected as target for the panning. A number of Fabs have been selected after five rounds of selection/amplification panning of the FDA2 library on gp120ΔV3$_{JRFL}$ and partially characterized. The CDR3 region of the heavy chains from positive clones

```
Ia3      AKPTYYDMLSGRSRHYYYMDV
Ia7      AAFRQWFGGLSGVFDS
II105    AKPSYYDMMSGRSRHYSYMDV
II116    DGSKWSRERKLFAPRARNFYYLD
Ia4      GPNERHWGSYRALYFES
Ib9      ASFRQWFGGLSGVFDS
II117    AAFDQWFGGLSGVYDS
```

Figure 5.3. CDR3 regions of Fabs selected from the panning of the FDA2 library with the gp120ΔV3 JRFL

were sequenced (Fig 5.3). Binding of these Fabs to both monomeric gp120 and trimeric gp120 on chronically infected cells was of high affinity as estimated by ELISA and flow cytometry. Fabs Ia7 and Ia3 neutralized HxB2 TCLA pseudotyped virus (Fig 5.4), but not PIs. Thus the most interesting Fab is probably Ia7 which has been further investigated. Fab Ia7 is directed against the CD4-BS on gp120 as it does compete for the binding of the virus to IgG1 b12 (data not shown).

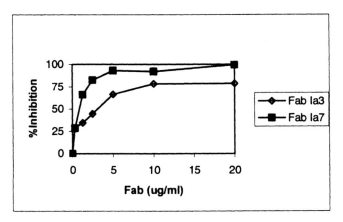

Figure 5.4. Neutralization of the HxB2 TCLA pseudotyped virus. HxB2, a TCLA virus was pseudotyped using the luciferase reporter assay and assayed for neutralization with Ia3 and Ia7 Fabs.

3.2   Antibodies Selected for Binding to gp120$_{JRFL}$-CD4-CCR5 Complexes

HIV enters cells by binding to receptor molecules (CD4 and coreceptors, mainly CCR5 and CXCR4) which induce conformational changes in the Env

(Dimitrov, 2000). We hypothesized that these conformational changes could enhance the exposure of conserved epitopes that might be targets for broadly neutralizing antibodies (Dimitrov, 1996; Moulard et al., 2002). The FDA2 library was panned on beads associated with CD4-gp120-CCR5 complexes. A gp120 specific Fab, X5, was selected after the fifth round of panning and was found to bind specifically to gp120 with high affinity (in the nanomolar range (Moulard et al., 2002)). Neutralization experiments demonstrated the potent and broad neutralizing activity of Fab X5 comparable to that of IgG1 b12 for more than 40 primary HIV isolates tested (Fig 5.5 and data not shown).

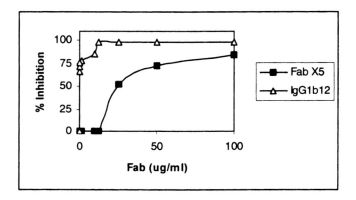

Figure 5.5. Neutralization of HIV-1HxB2 by the Fab X5 and IgG1b12. H9 cells were infected in the presence of IgG1b12 or Fab at indicated concentrations. Virus replication was assessed after 7 days by p24 ELISA measurement.

Recently, X5 was crystallized, its structure determined, and its epitope localized by molecular docking and alanine scanning mutagenesis (Xinhua et al., in preparation). The X5 epitope is located close proximity to the CD4 and coreceptor binding sites. The contact amino acid residues are highly conserved suggesting possible explanation for the breadth of neutralization.

3.3   Antibodies Selected by Sequential Antigen Panning (SAP)

We hypothesized that selection of high-affinity antibodies against conserved epitopes might be facilitated by sequentially changing the antigen during the panning of phage display libraries. We further hypothesized that the use of Env-CD4 complexes in combination with Envs alone as antigens may allow the identification of X5-like antibodies due to the highly conserved nature of the X5 epitope, the X5 high affinity binding to Env alone and its increased binding to Env-CD4 complexes. Five new HIV-specific antibodies (m12,14,16,18,20) were selected from an human Fab phage display library by using SAP against $gp140_{89.6}$–sCD4, $gp140_{IIIB}$-sCD4, $gp140_{89.6}$ and $gp140_{IIIB}$ followed by screening of individual clones with $gp140_{89.6}$, $gp120_{JR-FL}$ and $gp140_{IIIB}$, and their complexes with sCD4 (Zhang et al., in preparation). Some of these antibodies (m14 and m18) bound to Envs from several HIV isolates with high (nM) affinity, and inhibited virus entry and membrane fusion mediated by Envs of selected primary HIV isolates; the neutralization activity of these and other antibodies for a larger panel of isolates is being evaluated. The results suggest that the SAP is effective and could be used for identification of antibodies to conserved epitopes on rapidly mutating viruses or cells.

We used the same technology (SAP) in combination with random mutagenesis to further increase the breadth and potency of X5. Two scFvs (m6,9) were selected that exhibited several fold higher inhibitory activity to more than 30 primary HIV isolates compared to scFv and Fab X5 (Zhang et al., in preparation). These results may have implications for development of novel HIV inhibitors and vaccines.

4.   CONCLUSIONS

Phage display methodology has been successfully used for selection of high-affinity, potent, broadly HIV-1 nhmAbs. X5 binds to its epitope with an affinity that is enhanced by the Env interaction with CD4 but is not affected by CCR5; Fab X5 exhibits potent and broad neutralizing activity. The potency and breadth of X5 neutralizing activity was further enhanced by using random mutagenesis in combination with SAP; two scFvs, m6 and m9, selected by this approach exhibited higher neutralization activity than Fab and scFv X5. SAP was also used for selection of five new hmAb Fabs, two of which, m14 and m18, bind to epitopes close to the CD4 binding site, and three Fabs, m12, m16 and m20, bind to epitopes which are exposed better after the gp120 binding to CD4. The neutralizing activity of these antibodies is currently being evaluated. These results may have implications for development of novel HIV inhibitors and vaccines as well as for elucidation of the mechanisms of HIV entry into cells.

ACKNOWLEDGEMENTS

We are grateful to Prof. Dennis Burton for his comments which helped to significantly improve this article. We would like to thank all the colleagues who have helped in many invaluable ways to obtain the results presented in this chapter, in particular, the members of Drs. Burton and Dimitrov laboratories, and their collaborators. This project was partially supported by the NIH Intramural AIDS Targeted Antiviral Program (IATAP) and CPA from CCR, NCI to DSD, and DHHS #N01-C0-12400 to MYZ

REFERENCES

Armbruster,C., Stiegler,G.M., Vcelar,B.A., Jager,W., Michael,N.L., Vetter,N., and Katinger,H.W. (2002). A phase I trial with two human monoclonal antibodies (hMAb 2F5, 2G12) against HIV-1. AIDS *16*, 227-233.

Baba,T.W., Liska,V., Hofmann-Lehmann,R., Vlasak,J., Xu,W., Ayehunie,S., Cavacini,L.A., Posner,M.R., Katinger,H., Stiegler,G., Bernacky,B.J., Rizvi,T.A., Schmidt,R., Hill,L.R., Keeling,M.E., Lu,Y., Wright,J.E., Chou,T.C., and Ruprecht,R.M. (2000). Human neutralizing monoclonal antibodies of the IgG1 subtype protect against mucosal simian-human immunodeficiency virus infection. Nat. Med. *6*, 200-206.

Barbas,C.F., Burton,D.R., Scott,J.K., and Silverman,G.J. (2001). Phage Display: A Laboratory Mannual. (Cold Spring Harbor: Cold Spring Harbor Laboratory Press).

Barbas,C.F., III, Kang,A.S., Lerner,R.A., and Benkovic,S.J. (1991). Assembly of combinatorial antibody libraries on phage surfaces: the gene III site. Proc. Natl. Acad. Sci. U. S. A *88*, 7978-7982.

Bradbury,A., Persic,L., Werge,T., and Cattaneo,A. (1993). Use of living columns to select specific phage antibodies. Biotechnology (N. Y.) *11*, 1565-1569.

Burton,D.R. (1997). A vaccine for HIV type 1: the antibody perspective. Proc. Natl. Acad. Sci. U. S. A. *94*, 10018-10023.

Burton,D.R. (2002). Antibodies, viruses and vaccines. Nat. Rev. Immunol. *2*, 706-713.

Burton,D.R., Barbas,C.F., Persson,M.A., Koenig,S., Chanock,R.M., and Lerner,R.A. (1991). A large array of human monoclonal antibodies to type 1 human immunodeficiency virus from combinatorial libraries of asymptomatic seropositive individuals. Proc. Natl. Acad. Sci. U. S. A. *88*, 10134-10137.

Burton,D.R., Pyati,J., Koduri,R., Sharp,S.J., Thornton,G.B., Parren,P.W., Sawyer,L.S., Hendry,R.M., Dunlop,N., Nara,P.L., and et al. (1994). Efficient neutralization of primary isolates of HIV-1 by a recombinant human monoclonal antibody. Science *266*, 1024-1027.

Cai,X. and Garen,A. (1995). Anti-melanoma antibodies from melanoma patients immunized with genetically modified autologous tumor cells: selection of specific antibodies from single-chain Fv fusion phage libraries. Proc. Natl. Acad. Sci. U. S. A *92*, 6537-6541.

Clackson,T., Hoogenboom,H.R., Griffiths,A.D., and Winter,G. (1991). Making antibody fragments using phage display libraries. Nature *352*, 624-628.

de Kruif,J., Terstappen,L., Boel,E., and Logtenberg,T. (1995). Rapid selection of cell subpopulation-specific human monoclonal antibodies from a synthetic phage antibody library. Proc. Natl. Acad. Sci. U. S. A *92*, 3938-3942.

Dimitrov,D.S. (1996). Fusin - a place for HIV-1 and T4 cells to meet. Identifying the coreceptor mediating HIV-1 entry raises new hopes in the treatment of AIDS. Nature Medicine *2*, 640-641.

Dimitrov,D.S. (2000). Cell biology of virus entry. Cell. *101*, 697-702.

Ditzel,H.J. (2002). Rescue of a broader range of antibody specificities using an epitope-masking strategy. Methods Mol. Biol *178*, 179-186.

Ditzel,H.J., Binley,J.M., Moore,J.P., Sodroski,J., Sullivan,N., Sawyer,L.S., Hendry,R.M., Yang,W.P., Barbas,C.F., III, and Burton,D.R. (1995). Neutralizing recombinant human antibodies to a conformational V2- and CD4-binding site-sensitive epitope of HIV-1 gp120 isolated by using an epitope-masking procedure. J. Immunol. *154*, 893-906.

Ditzel,H.J., Masaki,Y., Nielsen,H., Farnaes,L., and Burton,D.R. (2000). Cloning and expression of a novel human antibody-antigen pair associated with Felty's syndrome. Proc. Natl. Acad. Sci. U. S. A. *97*, 9234-9239.

Duenas,M., Malmborg,A.C., Casalvilla,R., Ohlin,M., and Borrebaeck,C.A. (1996). Selection of phage displayed antibodies based on kinetic constants. Mol. Immunol. *33*, 279-285.

Ferrantelli,F. and Ruprecht,R.M. (2002). Neutralizing antibodies against HIV -- back in the major leagues? Curr. Opin. Immunol. *14*, 495-502.

Griffiths,A.D. and Duncan,A.R. (1998). Strategies for selection of antibodies by phage display. Curr. Opin. Biotechnol. *9*, 102-108.

Griffiths,A.D., Malmqvist,M., Marks,J.D., Bye,J.M., Embleton,M.J., McCafferty,J., Baier,M., Holliger,K.P., Gorick,B.D., Hughes-Jones,N.C., and . (1993). Human anti-self antibodies with high specificity from phage display libraries. EMBO J. *12*, 725-734.

Griffiths,A.D., Williams,S.C., Hartley,O., Tomlinson,I.M., Waterhouse,P., Crosby,W.L., Kontermann,R.E., Jones,P.T., Low,N.M., Allison,T.J., and . (1994). Isolation of high affinity human antibodies directly from large synthetic repertoires. EMBO J. *13*, 3245-3260.

Hallborn,J. and Carlsson,R. (2002). Automated screening procedure for high-throughput generation of antibody fragments. Biotechniques *Suppl*, 30-37.

Hawkins,R.E., Russell,S.J., and Winter,G. (1992). Selection of phage antibodies by binding affinity. Mimicking affinity maturation. J. Mol. Biol. *226*, 889-896.

Li,J., Pereira,S., Van Belle,P., Tsui,P., Elder,D., Speicher,D., Deen,K., Linnenbach,A., Somasundaram,R., Swoboda,R., and Herlyn,D. (2001). Isolation of the melanoma-associated antigen p23 using antibody phage display. J. Immunol. *166*, 432-438.

Marks,J.D., Hoogenboom,H.R., Bonnert,T.P., McCafferty,J., Griffiths,A.D., and Winter,G. (1991). By-passing immunization. Human antibodies from V-gene libraries displayed on phage. J. Mol. Biol *222*, 581-597.

Mascola,J.R. (2002). Passive transfer studies to elucidate the role of antibody-mediated protection against HIV-1. Vaccine *20*, 1922-1925.

Mascola,J.R., Lewis,M.G., Stiegler,G., Harris,D., VanCott,T.C., Hayes,D., Louder,M.K., Brown,C.R., Sapan,C.V., Frankel,S.S., Lu,Y., Robb,M.L., Katinger,H., and Birx,D.L. (1999). Protection of Macaques against pathogenic simian/human immunodeficiency virus 89.6PD by passive transfer of neutralizing antibodies. J. Virol. *73*, 4009-4018.

Mascola,J.R., Stiegler,G., VanCott,T.C., Katinger,H., Carpenter,C.B., Hanson,C.E., Beary,H., Hayes,D., Frankel,S.S., Birx,D.L., and Lewis,M.G. (2000). Protection of macaques against vaginal transmission of a pathogenic HIV- 1/SIV chimeric virus by passive infusion of neutralizing antibodies. Nat. Med. *6*, 207-210.

McCafferty,J., Griffiths,A.D., Winter,G., and Chiswell,D.J. (1990). Phage antibodies: filamentous phage displaying antibody variable domains. Nature *348*, 552-554.

Messmer,B.T. and Thaler,D.S. (2001). Specific blocking to improve biopanning in biological samples such as serum and hybridoma supernatants. Biotechniques *30*, 798-802.

Moreno,d.A., Martinez-alonso,C., Barbas,C.F., Burton,D.R., and Ditzel,H.J. (1995). Human monoclonal Fab fragments specific for viral antigens from combinatorial IgA libraries. Immunotechnology. *1*, 21-28.

Moulard,M., Lortat-Jacob,H., Mondor,I., Roca,G., Wyatt,R., Sodroski,J., Zhao,L., Olson,W., Kwong,P.D., and Sattentau,Q.J. (2000). Selective interactions of polyanions with basic surfaces on human immunodeficiency virus type 1 gp120. J. Virol. *74*, 1948-1960.

Moulard,M., Phogat,S.K., Shu,Y., Labrijn,A.F., Xiao,X., Binley,J.M., Zhang,M.Y., Sidorov,I.A., Broder,C.C., Robinson,J., Parren,P.W., Burton,D.R., and Dimitrov,D.S. (2002). Broadly cross-reactive HIV-1-neutralizing human monoclonal Fab selected for binding to gp120-CD4-CCR5 complexes. Proc. Natl. Acad. Sci. U. S. A *99*, 6913-6918.

Parren,P.W. and Burton,D.R. (1997). Antibodies against HIV-1 from phage display libraries: mapping of an immune response and progress towards antiviral immunotherapy. Chem. Immunol. *65*, 18-56.

Parren,P.W., Marx,P.A., Hessell,A.J., Luckay,A., Harouse,J., Cheng-Mayer,C., Moore,J.P., and Burton,D.R. (2001). Antibody protects macaques against vaginal challenge with a pathogenic R5 simian/human immunodeficiency virus at serum levels giving complete neutralization in vitro. J. Virol. *75*, 8340-8347.

Parren,P.W., Wang,M., Trkola,A., Binley,J.M., Purtscher,M., Katinger,H., Moore,J.P., and Burton,D.R. (1998). Antibody neutralization-resistant primary isolates of human immunodeficiency virus type 1. J. Virol. *72*, 10270-10274.

Poignard,P., Moulard,M., Golez,E., Vivona,V., Franti,M., Venturini,S., Wang,M., Parren,P.W., and Burton,D.R. (2003). Heterogeneity of envelope molecules expressed on primary human immunodeficiency virus type 1 particles as probed by the binding of neutralizing and nonneutralizing antibodies. J. Virol. *77*, 353-365.

Ruprecht,R.M., Hofmann-Lehmann,R., Smith-Franklin,B.A., Rasmussen,R.A., Liska,V., Vlasak,J., Xu,W., Baba,T.W., Chenine,A.L., Cavacini,L.A., Posner,M.R., Katinger,H., Stiegler,G., Bernacky,B.J., Rizvi,T.A., Schmidt,R., Hill,L.R., Keeling,M.E., Montefiori,D.C., and McClure,H.M. (2001). Protection of neonatal macaques against experimental SHIV infection by human neutralizing monoclonal antibodies. Transfus. Clin. Biol *8*, 350-358.

Sawyer,C., Embleton,J., and Dean,C. (1997). Methodology for selection of human antibodies to membrane proteins from a phage-display library. J. Immunol. Methods *204*, 193-203.

Schier,R., Balint,R.F., McCall,A., Apell,G., Larrick,J.W., and Marks,J.D. (1996a). Identification of functional and structural amino-acid residues by parsimonious mutagenesis. Gene *169*, 147-155.

Schier,R., Bye,J., Apell,G., McCall,A., Adams,G.P., Malmqvist,M., Weiner,L.M., and Marks,J.D. (1996b). Isolation of high-affinity monomeric human anti-c-erbB-2 single chain Fv using affinity-driven selection. J. Mol. Biol. *255*, 28-43.

Schier,R. and Marks,J.D. (1996). Efficient in vitro affinity maturation of phage antibodies using BIAcore guided selections. Hum. Antibodies Hybridomas *7*, 97-105.

Schier,R., McCall,A., Adams,G.P., Marshall,K.W., Merritt,H., Yim,M., Crawford,R.S., Weiner,L.M., Marks,C., and Marks,J.D. (1996c). Isolation of picomolar affinity anti-c-erbB-2 single-chain Fv by molecular evolution of the complementarity determining regions in the center of the antibody binding site. J. Mol. Biol. *263*, 551-567.

Shibata,R., Igarashi,T., Haigwood,N., Buckler-White,A., Ogert,R., Ross,W., Willey,R., Cho,M.W., and Martin,M.A. (1999). Neutralizing antibody directed against the HIV-1 envelope glycoprotein can completely block HIV-1/SIV chimeric virus infections of macaque monkeys. Nat. Med. *5*, 204-210.

Stiegler,G., Armbruster,C., Vcelar,B., Stoiber,H., Kunert,R., Michael,N.L., Jagodzinski,L.L., Ammann,C., Jager,W., Jacobson,J., Vetter,N., and Katinger,H. (2002). Antiviral activity of the neutralizing antibodies 2F5 and 2G12 in asymptomatic HIV-1-infected humans: a phase I evaluation. AIDS *16*, 2019-2025.

Toran,J.L., Kremer,L., Sanchez-Pulido,L., de Alboran,I.M., del Real,G., Llorente,M., Valencia,A., de Mon,M.A., and Martinez,A. (1999). Molecular analysis of HIV-1 gp120 antibody response using isotype IgM and IgG phage display libraries from a long-term non-progressor HIV-1- infected individual. Eur. J. Immunol. *29*, 2666-2675.

Trepel,M., Arap,W., and Pasqualini,R. (2002). In vivo phage display and vascular heterogeneity: implications for targeted medicine. Curr. Opin. Chem. Biol. *6*, 399-404.

Van Ewijk,W., de Kruif,J., Germeraad,W.T., Berendes,P., Ropke,C., Platenburg,P.P., and Logtenberg,T. (1997). Subtractive isolation of phage-displayed single-chain antibodies to thymic stromal cells by using intact thymic fragments. Proc. Natl. Acad. Sci. U. S. A *94*, 3903-3908.

Veazey,R.S., Shattock,R.J., Pope,M., Kirijan,J.C., Jones,J., Hu,Q., Ketas,T., Marx,P.A., Klasse,P.J., Burton,D.R., and Moore,J.P. (2003). Prevention of virus transmission to macaque monkeys by a vaginally applied monoclonal antibody to HIV-1 gp120. Nat. Med. *9*, 343-346.

Vujcic,L.K. and Quinnan,G.V., Jr. (1995). Preparation and characterization of human HIV type 1 neutralizing reference sera. AIDS Res. Hum. Retroviruses *11*, 783-787.

Williams,B.R., Sompuram,S.R., and Sharon,J. (2002). Generation of anti-colorectal cancer fab phage display libraries with a high percentage of diverse antigen-reactive clones. Comb. Chem. High Throughput. Screen. *5*, 489-499.

Williamson,R.A., Burioni,R., Sanna,P.P., Partridge,L.J., Barbas,C.F., III, and Burton,D.R. (1993a). Human monoclonal antibodies against a plethora of viral pathogens from single combinatorial libraries. Proc. Natl. Acad. Sci. U. S. A *90*, 4141-4145.

Williamson,R.A., Burioni,R., Sanna,P.P., Partridge,L.J., Barbas,C.F., and Burton,D.R. (1993b). Human monoclonal antibodies against a plethora of viral pathogens from single combinatorial libraries [published erratum appears in Proc Natl Acad Sci U S A 1994 Feb 1;91(3):1193]. Proc. Natl. Acad. Sci. U. S. A. *90*, 4141-4145.

Xu,W., Hofmann-Lehmann,R., McClure,H.M., and Ruprecht,R.M. (2002). Passive immunization with human neutralizing monoclonal antibodies: correlates of protective immunity against HIV. Vaccine *20*, 1956-1960.

Zwick,M.B., Bonnycastle,L.L., Menendez,A., Irving,M.B., Barbas,C.F., III, Parren,P.W., Burton,D.R., and Scott,J.K. (2001a). Identification and Characterization of a Peptide That Specifically Binds the Human, Broadly Neutralizing Anti-Human Immunodeficiency Virus Type 1 Antibody b12. J. Virol. *75*, 6692-6699.

Zwick,M.B., Labrijn,A.F., Wang,M., Spenlehauer,C., Saphire,E.O., Binley,J.M., Moore,J.P., Stiegler,G., Katinger,H., Burton,D.R., and Parren,P.W. (2001b). Broadly neutralizing antibodies targeted to the membrane-proximal external region of human immunodeficiency virus type 1 glycoprotein gp41. J. Virol. *75*, 10892-10905.

Chapter 6

MONOCLONAL AND BISPECIFIC ANTIBODIES IN COMBINATION WITH RADIOTHERAPY FOR CANCER TREATMENT

David Azria[1,2], Christel Larbouret[1], Bruno Robert[1], Mahmut Ozsahin[3], Jean-Bernard Dubois[1,2], André Pèlegrin[1]

[1] *Immunociblage des Tumeurs et Ingénierie des Anticorps, EMI 0227 INSERM-Université Montpellier I-CRLC Montpellier, Centre de Recherche en Cancérologie, CRLC Val d'Aurelle – Paul Lamarque, F-34298 Montpellier Cedex 5, France ;* [2] *Department of Radiation Oncology, CRLC Val d'Aurelle - Paul Lamarque, F-34298 Montpellier Cedex 5, France ;* [3] *Department of Radiation Oncology, Centre Hospitalier Universitaire Vaudois, CH-1011 Lausanne, Suisse*

1.   INTRODUCTION

In recent years, the advent of new tumor-targeting vectors such as monoclonal or bispecific antibodies has resulted in the development of a new generation of therapeutic radiopharmaceuticals and an increasing research interest in this field. However, the emphasis in the overwhelming majority of such studies has been on efficacy in clinical conditions or in animal models of human cancers, and little consideration has been given to the effects of the combination of these antibodies and radiation therapy.

The cell membrane has been known for some time to be a secondary target for ionizing radiation. It is also the source of cytokine receptors, such as those for epidermal growth factor (EGF) and tumor necrosis factor (TNF). These may be activated by ionizing radiation, thus provoking the pathways of mitogen-activated protein kinase (MAPK), phosphatidyl inositol-3-phosphate kinase (PI3K), and MAPK8 activation (Schmidt-Ullrich et al., 2000), which can modulate cell proliferation or death.

TNFα is a multipotent cytokine produced mainly by activated macrophages. It was originally identified as a tumoricidal protein effecting hemorrhagic necrosis of transplanted solid tumors in mice (Carswell et al., 1975) but it has since been implicated in diverse biological processes including inflammation and immunoregulation, antiviral defense, endotoxic shock, cachexia, angiogenesis, and mitogenesis (Beutler & Cerami, 1988; Old, 1988). In addition to this wide range of biological activities is the ability to mediate cytotoxicity both *in vitro* (Sugarman et al., 1985) and *in vivo* (Carswell et al., 1975; Helson et al., 1979). The oxidative damage produced by TNFα may enhance cellular damage produced by ionizing radiation. The consistent use of a bispecific antibody to concentrate TNFα into tumors was the basis of our variety of works for radiosensitization with TNFα, and all the data are developed in part one of the present chapter.

Preclinical and clinical studies associate EGF receptors overexpression with radioresistance (Balaban et al., 1996; Barker et al., 2001; Gupta et al., 2002; Wollman et al., 1994). Consistent with the variety of mechanisms of EGF Receptors family member dysregulation, several approaches have been used for inhibition of these receptors. Cetuximab (Erbitux®) is an anti-EGFR antibody that blocks binding of EGF ligands to the EGFR, inhibiting EGFR activation, particularly activation because of autocrine stimulation (Baselga, 2001). Trastuzumab (Herceptin®) is an anti-HER2 antibody. Although the mechanism of action is not entirely clear, the preponderance of evidence suggests that Herceptin® binds to HER2 homodimers that occur when HER2 is overexpressed to the high levels seen with gene amplification, and accelerates downregulation of the receptors (Klapper et al., 1997). Investigations of the radiation response modulation by the EGF receptors inhibitors are described in the second part of this chapter.

2.   BISPECIFIC ANTIBODIES, CYTOKINES AND RADIATION THERAPY

Efficient targeting and site specific actions of tumor therapeutics represent a major challenge in oncology, in particular for cytokine based therapeutic strategies because of their typically pleiotropic actions throughout the body. Antibody-directed targeting of cytokines is a promising first step to improve therapeutic efficacy and to limit their systemic side-effects after intravenous injections.

In 1996, we evaluated the capability of a bispecific antibody (BAb) directed against carcinoembryonic antigen (CEA) and human tumor necrosis factor alpha (TNFα) to target this cytokine in tumors (Robert et al., 1996) (Figure 6.1). A BAb was constructed by coupling the Fab' fragments from an anti-CEA monoclonal antibody (MAb) to the Fab' fragments from an anti-TNFα MAb via a stable thioether linkage. The double specificity of the BAb for CEA and TNFα was demonstrated using a BIAcore™ two-step analysis. The affinity constants of the BAb for CEA immobilized on a sensor chip and for soluble TNFα added to the CEA-BAb complex were as high as those of the parental MAbs $(1.7 \times 10^9 \, M^{-1}$ and $6.6 \times 10^8 \, M^{-1}$, respectively). The

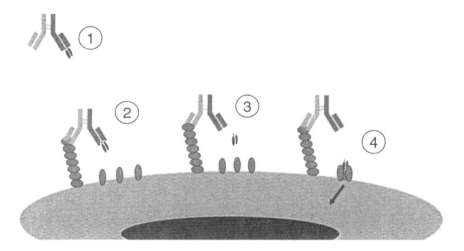

Figure 6.1. Bispecific antibodies (BAb) for cytokine targeting. 1/ BAb is composed with an arm directed against a tumor associated antigen (eg CEA) and one arm directed against the cytokine (eg TNFα). The BAb and the cytokine are pre-incubated before injection in the organism. 2/ The BAb-cytokine complex is targeted on CEA expressing tumor cells. 3/ TNFα can "jump" from the BAb to its receptor. 4/ Following binding on its receptor, TNFα can produce its whole physiological activity. Adapted from (Robert et al., 1996).

radiolabeled ^{125}I-labeled BAb retained high immunoreactivity with both CEA and TNFα immobilized on a solid phase. In nude mice xenografted with the human colorectal carcinoma T380, the ^{125}I-labeled BAb showed a tumor localization and biodistribution comparable to that of ^{131}I-labeled anti-CEA parental F(ab')$_2$ with 25-30% of the injected dose (ID)/g tumor at 24 h and 20% ID/g tumor at 48 h. To target TNFα in the tumor, a two-step i.v. injection protocol was used first, in which a variable dose of ^{125}I-labeled BAb was injected, followed 24 or 48 h later by a constant dose of ^{131}I-labeled TNFα (1 μg). Mice pretreated with 3 μg of BAb and sacrificed 2, 4, 6, or 8 h after the injection of TNFα showed a 1.5- to 2-fold increased concentration of ^{131}I-labeled TNFα in the tumor as compared to control mice receiving TNFα alone. With a higher dose of BAb (25 µg), mice showed a better targeting of TNFα with a 3.2-fold increased concentration of ^{131}I-labeled TNFα in the tumor: 9.3% versus 2.9% ID/g in control mice 6 h after TNFα injection. In a one-step injection protocol using a premixed BAb-TNFα preparation, similar results were obtained 6 h post-injection (3.5-fold increased TNFα tumor concentration). A longer retention time of TNFα was observed leading to an 8.1-fold increased concentration of TNFα in the tumor 14 h postinjection (4.4 versus 0.5% ID/g tumor for BAb-treated and control mice, respectively). These results showed that our BAb was able to localize in a human colon carcinoma and, therefore, to immunoabsorb the i.v.-injected TNFα, leading to its increased concentration at the tumor site.

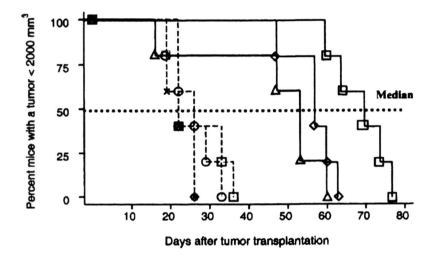

Days after tumor transplantation

Figure 6 2. Kaplan-Meier survival curves obtained as a function of time for all groups: Group 1: Dotted line (**X**) no treatment (22 days); Group 2: Dotted line (◊) TNFα (22 days); Group 3: Dotted line (○) BAb (26 days); Group 4: Dotted line (□) BAb + TNFα (22 days); Group 5: Solid line (Δ) RT (57 days); Group 6: Solid line (◊) RT + TNFα (61 days); Group 7: Solid line (□) RT + TNFα + BAb (67 days). All mice were sacrificed when the xeno-transplants reached this volume. The number in parentheses corresponds to the median delay (time taken for the tumor to reach a volume of 2000 mm³ in 50% of the mice). Reproduced with permission from (Azria et al., 2003a).

More recently, we co-injected this BAb with TNFα in pre-clinical models to enhance radiation tumor responses (Azria et al., 2003a). It has been known for many years that TNFα interacts with radiation to enhance killing of some human tumor cell lines *in vitro* with additive or synergistic effect at a TNFα concentration that produces cytotoxicity in 10% of cells (Hallahan et al., 1990). In our study, we found that TNFα enhanced significantly radiation-induced cell death in several digestive tumor cells, particularly if cells were very sensitive to TNFα used alone (Azria et al., 2003b). Our experimental results were plotted within the envelope of additivity near the mode II line and demonstrated a simple additive effect of the combination. In addition, the isobologram analysis suggests that radiotherapy (RT) and TNFα act in the same way either in colon cancer model (LS174T) or in the pancreatic cell line (BxPC-3).

In vivo, in LS174T and BxPC-3 xenografts, RT as a single agent slowed tumor progression as compared to control group. In LS174T model, TNFα-RT combination enhanced the delay to reach 2000 mm^3 as compared to RT alone but with no statistical difference. This delay was significantly longer when BAb was added (Figure 6.2). In BxPC-3 experiments, median delay to reach 2000 mm^3 was similar between RT and TNFα-RT groups. The use of our BAb in combination with TNFα and RT dramatically enhanced this median delay (Figure 6.3).

Because of the pleiotropic effect of TNFα, the effects of TNFα on the immune system must be considered. These studies will be performed in an immunocompetent animal model. However, many published data concerning nude mice experiments have shown that TNFα and RT may enhance the therapeutic efficacy of RT in tumor xenograft models (Gridley et al., 1997; Gridley et al., 1994; Nishiguchi et al., 1990; Sersa et al., 1988). These results support the fact that *in vivo* interactions between TNFα and RT may also be explained by nonimmunological phenomenon such as the involvement of endothelial cell integrin αvβ3 in the disruption of the tumor vasculature by TNFα (Ruegg et al., 1998) that could further promote RT local action. Nevertheless, we did not show significant improvement of TNFα and RT combination as compared to RT alone in our models (LS174T and BxPC-3 xenografts) probably due in part to a poor tumor uptake of free injected TNFα. These results reinforce our hypothesis that an anti-CEA/anti-TNFα BAb can concentrate TNFα in a CEA-expressing tumor to improve RT and finally to keep a large differential effect between tumor and normal tissues.

Our data could be used as a solid preclinical rationale on which to base a clinical study in locally advanced pancreatic cancers in the near future. The use of a chimeric or a humanized bispecific antibody anti-CEA/anti-TNFα will reduce the risk of development of human anti-murine antibody (HAMA) reaction.

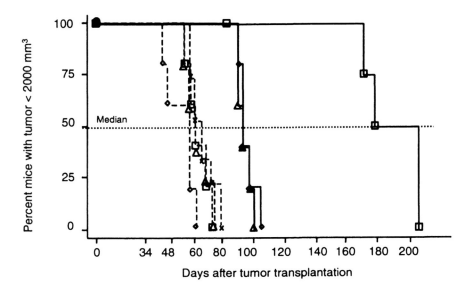

Figure 6.3. Kaplan-Meier survival curves obtained as a function of time for all groups: Group 1: Dotted line (O) no treatment (65 days); Group 2: Dotted line (◊) TNFα (62 days); Group 3: Dotted line (**X**) BAb (72 days); Group 4: Dotted line (□) BAb + TNFα (65 days); Group 5: Solid line (Δ) RT (93 days); Group 6: Solid line (◊) RT + TNFα (93 days); Group 7: Solid line (□) RT + TNFα + BAb (177 days). All mice were sacrificed when the xeno-transplants reached a volume of 2000 mm³. The number in parentheses corresponds to the median delay (time taken for the tumor to reach a volume of 2000 mm³ in 50% of the mice). Adapted from Azria et al, 2004.

3. MONOCLONAL ANTIBODIES AGAINST EPIDERMAL GROWTH FACTOR RECEPTORS: RADIATION RESPONSE MODULATORS

Growing evidence suggests that epidermal growth factor (EGF) family (HER) receptors play a significant role in radiation response. Promising results have been obtained in experimental studies assessing the combined use of EGF receptor inhibitors and RT. Based on these data, a number of clinical trials were started.

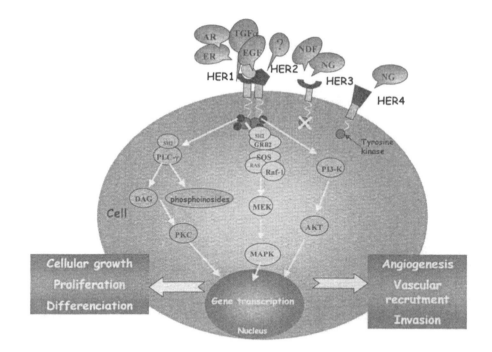

Figure 6.4. Intra-cellular signalization network of HER family receptors: AR, amphiregulin; ER, epiregulin; TGFα, tumor growth factor alpha; EGF, epidermal growth factor; NDF,neu differentiation factor; NG, neuregulin; PLC-γ, phospholipase C γ; DAG, diacylglycerol; PKC, protein kinase C; GRB, growth factor receptor bound protein; SOS, son of sevenless; MEK, mitogen-activated-protein/extracellular signal-regulated kinase; MAPK, mitogen-activated protein kinase; PI3-K, phosphatidyl inositol-3-phosphate kinase; AKT, protein kinase B.

3.1 EGF receptor family (or HER)

Four transmembrane EGF receptors are known: HER1/EGFR, HER2, HER3, and HER4 (Carpenter & Cohen, 1990). HER1 and HER2 are increasingly used as therapeutic targets in association with ionizing radiation.

These receptors have three domains: (i) an extracellular domain, which is situated at the aminoterminal end permitting the detection and fixation of a specific ligand; (ii) a transmembrane hydrophobe domain, which realizes the anchoring of receptor in the cell membrane; and (iii) an intracytoplasmic domain, which includes an enzymatic tyrosine kinase containing the fixation sites of ATP and proteic substrates to be phosphorylated, and a carboxy-terminal domain regulating the receptor activity and autophosphorylation (van der Geer et al., 1994; Yarden & Ullrich, 1988).

HER1 and HER2 exist in chemically inactive monomer form or in chemically active dimer form. Dimerization can take place between different receptors in order to develop homologue (homodimers) or heterologue (heterodimers) dimers (Alroy & Yarden, 1997). The tyrosine kinase site of the HER3 receptor does not seem to be active (Guy et al., 1994). Several ligands have been described, and they create a cascade of intracellular signals following fixation on their respective receptors. Transforming growth factor α (TGFα) seems to be the most common ligand among the six described ones (TGFα, EGF, β-cellulin, epiregulin, amphiregulin, and heparin-binding EGF). To our knowledge, no ligand could be identified for the HER2 receptor (Yarden, 2001). Transduction signals are created after fixation of respective ligands, and dimerization of the receptors are developed by autophosphorylation of intracellular tyrosine-dependent catalytic domain. Residual phosphorylated tyrosine becomes an anchoring point for several cytoplasmic protein domains such as SH2, Src homology domain 2 (Tse et al., 1997).

Proteins like phospholipase C-γ (PLC-γ), phosphatidylinositol-3'-kinase (PI-3K), GTPase activating protein (GAP), and SH2 containing protein (SHC) surround activated receptors and, therefore, induce intracellular signal cascades where intermediate proteins like Ras, Raf, and mitogen-activated protein kinase (MAPK) are involved (Chen et al., 1998; Franke et al., 1997; Hynes & Stern, 1994; Janes et al., 1994; Ram & Ethier, 1996; Ullrich & Schlessinger, 1990). In a normal cell, EGF receptor activity is strictly regulated via positive and negative stimulation signals (Moghal & Sternberg, 1999). In cancer cells, numerous mechanisms can activate the PI-3K or MAPK pathways such as (i) receptor overexpression, (ii) increased ligand concentration, (iii) decreased phosphatase activity, and (iv) presence of abnormal receptors such as EGFRvIII, which prevents the fixation of ligands (Moscatello et al., 1998; Voldborg et al., 1997). In either normal or malignant cells, the activation of EGF receptor cascades may have multiple consequences. Cell growth, differentiation, and proliferation are stimulated by the activation of nuclear proteins such as cyclin D1, which regulates the passage from the G1 phase to the S phase (Perry et al., 1998). The inhibition of cellular proliferation by an anti-EGF monoclonal antibody is characterized by a G1 arrest and, therefore, induction of apoptosis (Wu et al., 1995; Wu et al., 1996). The cellular differentiation and/or proliferation capacity depends not only on the cell type but also on the intensity and the duration of activation of the MAPK transduction pathway. Thus, a short activation of cellular growth factors results with an increase in cellular proliferation via increased cyclin D1 expression and, therefore, progression towards the G2/M phase. However, paradoxally, prolonged exposition to the same growth factors results with decreased DNA synthesis. This latter is probably related to the induction of p21$^{CIP-1/WAFI}$, a protein responsible for the G1 arrest in the cell cycle (Auer et al., 1998; Tombes et al., 1998).

EGF receptor cascades may also promote malignant transformation, angiogenesis, and/or metastatic dissemination (Allred et al., 1992; Hudziak et al., 1987). Malignant cells escape the inhibition of proliferation process by the overexpression of EGF receptor family members; e.g., when HER2 is overexpressed, its activation is possible via dimerization and autoactivation, even without any stimulus (Di Fiore et al., 1987; Ignatoski et al., 1999). This overexpression is characterized by uncontrolled cell proliferation and malignant transformation, including either *in vitro* colony forming capacity or development of new tumors in nude mice (Bishop, 1991; Dougall et al., 1994; Lin et al., 1995).

The use of anti-EGF-R antibodies results in decreased VEGF expression in culture and *in vivo*, and reduction in tumor growth (Perrotte et al., 1999). An increased level and/or activity of EGFR and HER2 seem to increase the metastatic potential of malignant cells (Allred et al., 1992; Radinsky et al., 1995). Limited clinical experience revealed that overexpression of HER1 or HER2 in tumors resulted in increased local recurrence rate, decreased overall and disease-free survival, and increased lymph node infiltration (Berger et al., 1988; Nicholson et al., 2001). HER1 or HER2 receptor blockage using monoclonal antibodies has been shown to be efficient in terms of decreased metastatic potential in a number of animal (Naramura et al., 1993; Zolfaghari & Djakiew, 1996) and human studies (Cobleigh et al., 1999).

3.2 Monoclonal antibodies as HER1 and HER2 inhibitors

There is an increasing number of experimental and clinical evidence that EGF receptor family members or their ligands constitute an important target in the treatment of cancer. The use of EGF receptor inhibitors such as monoclonal antibodies (MAb) seems to be promising.

MAbs bind generally the extracellular domain of the EGF receptor, and block the fixation of the ligand to its receptor and, therefore, intracellular signalling cascade (Baselga & Albanell, 2001; Ciardiello & Tortora, 2001; Slichenmyer & Fry, 2001). At present, a number of MAbs are used in the experimental and clinical studies (Slichenmyer & Fry, 2001). Among them, only Trastuzumab (Herceptin®) and Cetuximab (Erbitux®) are used in preclinical or clinical studies together with radiation therapy.

3.2.1   Cetuximab (Erbitux®)

Cetuximab (Erbitux®) is a chimeric monoclonal antibody obtained by replacing the constant domains of the 225 murine monoclonal antibody by those of a human IgG1 (Goldstein et al., 1995; Naramura et al., 1993). This structure was developed in order to produce significantly less anti-murine human antibodies. Cetuximab, by blocking specifically HER1, prevents ligand fixation, receptor heterodimerization, and intracellular signal activation (Huang & Harari, 1999). Cetuximab inhibits cellular proliferation, promotes apoptosis and G1 phase arrest (Huang et al., 1999; Peng et al., 1996; Wu et al., 1995). It also inhibits angiogenesis (Perrotte et al., 1999; Petit et al., 1997), therefore, metastatic potential (Naramura et al., 1993; Perrotte et al., 1999). A number of preclinical animal studies demonstrated encouraging results in terms of volume decrease in tumor xenotransplants (Aboud-Pirak et al., 1988; Prewett et al., 1998; Schnurch et al., 1994; Teramoto et al., 1996), which permitted the start-up of several phase I-II human studies using Cetuximab as monotherapy or in combination with other chemotherapeutic agents (Baselga, 2001; Baselga et al., 2000).

3.2.2   Trastuzumab (Herceptin®)

Trastuzumab, a humanized antibody, is a result of the combination of a human IgG1 (95%) and the HER2 antigen binding site of the murine 4D5 (5%) antibody (Carter et al., 1992). Antitumoral activity of trastuzumab, alone or in combination with other drugs, has been largely reported in preclinical studies (Baselga et al., 1998; Tokuda et al., 1996). Trastuzumab (i) permits receptor homodimerization and autophosphorylation without activating intracellular signals, and this first step could have a negative feedback effect on the number of HER2 receptors on the cellular membrane (Sliwkowski et al., 1999); (ii) prevents the formation of HER2-HER3 and HER2-HER4 heterodimers (Klapper et al., 1997); (iii) promotes actively G1 phase cell cycle arrest by the induction of p27 protein (Lane et al., 2001; Sliwkowski et al., 1999), and shortens the S phase (Sliwkowski et al., 1999); (iv) inhibits angiogenesis (Izumi et al., 2002; Petit et al., 1997); and (v) induces antibody-dependent cellular cytotoxicity (ADCC) (Clynes et al., 2000), activates the complement (Jurianz et al., 1999) and, therefore, stimulates the HER2-specific class I cytotoxic activity of CD8 T-lymphocytes (zum Buschenfelde et al., 2002).

Several phase I and II clinical studies assessed the pharmacokinetics, the toxicity, the maximal tolerable dose, and the efficacy of trastuzumab in metastatic breast cancer patients (Baselga et al., 1996; Cobleigh et al., 1999; Pegram et al., 1998; Shak, 1999). A recently published phase III study revealed the beneficial effect of trastuzumab as a first line treatment combined with chemotherapy in metastatic breast cancer (Slamon et al., 2001).

3.3   Anti-HER1 and –HER2 MAbs and radiotherapy

Ionizing radiation produces several types of cellular response via activation of multiple transduction pathways resulting with cell death, differentiation, or proliferation. This response depends mainly on cell type, irradiation dose, or cell-culture conditions (Carter et al., 1998; Chmura et al., 1997; Haimovitz-Friedman, 1998; Kavanagh et al., 1998; Santana et al., 1996; Schmidt-Ullrich et al., 1997; Xia et al., 1995). Following irradiation, the MAPK pathway was recently reported to be a cellular "SOS" signal initiator starting from EGF receptors (Schmidt-Ullrich et al., 1997). MAPK pathway activation via HER1 receptors was reported in many malignant human cell lines (Carter et al., 1998; Kavanagh et al., 1998; Schmidt-Ullrich et al., 1997). This activation is similar to the one produced by physiological concentrations of EGF (0.1 nM), and seems to act as a radioprotector (Balaban et al., 1996; Goldkorn et al., 1997; Kavanagh et al., 1998; Schmidt-Ullrich et al., 1997). The activation of MAPK pathway includes also the activation of phospholipase γ (PLCγ) and protein kinase C (PKC)/Ras/Raf complex (Dent et al., 1995; Ghosh et al., 1996; Marais et al., 1995). Moreover, MAPK activation following ionizing radiation have many consequences which can be contradictory. The ability of cell-cycle G2 arrest inhibition following irradiation depends on MAPK cascade activation, and seems to be superior when cells express high levels of RAF1 proto-oncogene (Abbott & Holt, 1999; Warenius et al., 1996). This decrease in radiation-induced G2 arrest would authorize the passage of many cells with DNA damage into mitosis and, therefore, a loss in their clonogenic potential. Furthermore, an increase in radiation-induced p21$^{CIP-1/WAF1}$ protein, and a transitory G1 arrest were recently reported to be related to the same activation pathway resulting with a slow-down in cell-cycle progression and, therefore, DNA repair (Carter et al., 1998). These findings support the positive and negative role of MAPK signal pathway following irradiation in the down regulation of cell cycle in cancer cells. The conversion of a radioresistant cell phenotype to a more radiosensible phenotype is reported in a glial tumor cell-line transformed by functional inhibition of the MAPK signalization pathway (O'Rourke et al., 1998). Moreover, it has been recently shown that EGF-receptor and MAPK signal pathway activation following ionizing radiation depends on the proteolytic clivage of TGFα precursor and functional activation of autocrine TGFα (Dent et al., 1999).

STAT-3 signal pathway activation by phosphorylation via EGF receptors can be initiated by ionizing radiation, and it results with a radioprotective effect by apoptosis inhibition (David et al., 1996; Grandis et al., 2000; Park et al., 1996). The use of Cetuximab (1 µg/ml) alone or combined with radiation therapy (4 Gy) results with a major reduction in phosphorylated STAT-3 and, therefore, an augmentation of apoptosis (Bonner et al., 2000b).

An inverse relation between the number of EGF receptors and tumor radiocurability is reported in several murine cell lines. In these models, radiation-induced apoptosis was decreased when important levels of EGF receptor were expressed on the cells (Akimoto et al., 1999). Clinical consequences of these findings would be tailoring treatment according to a simple predictive assay of radiosensitivity based on the EGF-receptor expression. Moreover, tumor repopulation between the two fractions of radiation therapy may be considered as a consequence of EGF-receptor activation (Schmidt-Ullrich et al., 1997) and, therefore, would be depending on inhibitor agents such as anti-EGF-R monoclonal antibodies.

3.3.1 Cetuximab (Erbitux®) and radiotherapy

Based on the radiobiological issues discussed above, the association of radiation therapy and Cetuximab was tested in several *in vitro* and *in vivo* studies (Bianco et al., 2000; Huang & Harari, 1999; Huang & Harari, 2000; Milas et al., 2000; Saleh et al., 1999).

Cetuximab inhibits radiation-induced sublethal or potentially lethal damage repair in squamous-cell carcinoma cell lines derived from human oropharyngeal cancer (SCC-13Y, SCC-1, and SCC-6). This inhibition is a consequence of the nuclear reduction in DNA-PK (enzyme functioning in the complex multiproteic repair of radiation-induced lesions) (Huang & Harari, 2000).

In vivo, the association of Cetuximab with radiation therapy decreases not only the expression of several factors active in angiogenesis, i.e. VEGF, but also the diameter of small vessels (Huang & Harari, 2000). Several data on different animal models (squamous-cell carcinoma of the oropharynx, adenocarcinoma of the colon or ovaries) confirmed significant reduction of tumor volume following xenografts on nude mice in the groups using the combination of Cetuximab and radiation therapy (Bianco et al., 2000; Buchsbaum et al., 2002; Huang & Harari, 2000; Milas et al., 2000; Nasu et al., 2001; Saleh et al., 1999).

The first phase I/II clinical studies are actually on-going. Bonner *et al* (Bonner et al., 2000a) presented in an abstract form one of the first phase I/II clinical trials including 15 patients with head and neck squamous-cell carcinoma. In this study, RT was delivered using either standard fractionation (70 Gy / 35 fractions / 7 weeks) or hyperfractionated RT (74.4 Gy/62 fractions/7 weeks). By progressively increasing the Cetuximab dose, the maximum tolerable dose (MTD) was found to be 400 mg/m^2 as an induction dose, and the maintenance dose 250 mg/m^2/week (Bonner et al., 2000b). The authors obtained 13 complete and 2 partial responses out of 15 patients. After two years 9 of 15 patients were still locoregionally controlled (Bonner et al., 2000a). Because of these encouraging results, a phase III study comparing RT alone and RT + Cetuximab was conducted between 1999 and 2001. Final results will not be published before late 2004.

3.3.2   Trastuzumab (Herceptin®) and radiotherapy

Trastuzumab has been tested in combination with RT on a breast cancer cell line with important HER2 expression (MCF-7/HER2) (Pietras et al., 1999). This association permits, using an *in vitro* clonogenic assay, to radiosensitize this cell line known to be relatively resistant. Radiosensitization is thought to be a consequence of decreased DNA-repair capacity of radiation-induced lesions by Trastuzumab. *In vivo* studies showed that by transplanting these tumor cells to nude mice, the use of Trastuzumab (3 injections of 30 mg/kg 4 h after RT) together with RT (4x4 Gy) decreased significantly tumor progression (Pietras et al., 1999). Similar *in vitro* results have been obtained on other cell lines of head and neck or ovarian origin (Schmidt et al., 2001; Stackhouse et al., 1998; Uno et al., 2001).

4.   CONCLUSION

Monoclonal antibodies against members of the EGFR family and bispecific antibodies targeting cytokines such as TNFα constitute attractive biological response modifiers which can be combined to radiotherapy. Future studies could make a bridge between these two families of molecules based on the results obtained by (i) Hudziak et al. demonstrating that anti-HER2 MAbs sensitize human breast cancer cells to TNFα (Hudziak et al., 1989) and (ii) Hambek et al. who demonstrated using 1060 different xenotransplants that TNFα sensitizes low EGFR-expressing carcinomas for anti-EGFR MAb therapy (Hambek et al., 2001).

Combination of these antibodies with conventional therapies such as radiation is an evidence that they are now filling a growing place in the treatment of cancer patients.

REFERENCES

Abbott, D.W. & Holt, J.T. (1999). Mitogen-activated protein kinase kinase 2 activation is essential for progression through the G2/M checkpoint arrest in cells exposed to ionizing radiation. *J Biol Chem*, **274**, 2732-42.

Aboud-Pirak, E., Hurwitz, E., Pirak, M.E., Bellot, F., Schlessinger, J. & Sela, M. (1988). Efficacy of antibodies to epidermal growth factor receptor against KB carcinoma in vitro and in nude mice. *J Natl Cancer Inst*, **80**, 1605-11.

Akimoto, T., Hunter, N.R., Buchmiller, L., Mason, K., Kian Ang, K. & Milas, L. (1999). Inverse relationship between epidermal growth factor receptor expression and radiocurability of murine carcinomas. *Clin Cancer Res*, **5**, 2884-2890.

Allred, D.C., Clark, G.M., Molina, R., Tandon, A.K., Schnitt, S.J., Gilchrist, K.W., Osborne, C.K., Tormey, D.C. & McGuire, W.L. (1992). Overexpression of HER-2/neu and its relationship with other prognostic factors change during the progression of in situ to invasive breast cancer. *Hum Pathol*, **23**, 974-9.

Alroy, I. & Yarden, Y. (1997). The ErbB signaling network in embryogenesis and oncogenesis: signal diversification through combinatorial ligand-receptor interactions. *FEBS Lett*, **410**, 83-6.

Auer, K.L., Park, J.S., Seth, P., Coffey, R.J., Darlington, G., Abo, A., McMahon, M., Depinho, R.A., Fisher, P.B. & Dent, P. (1998). Prolonged activation of the mitogen-activated protein kinase pathway promotes DNA synthesis in primary hepatocytes from p21Cip-1/WAF1-null mice, but not in hepatocytes from p16INK4a-null mice. *Biochem J*, **336**, 551-60.

Azria, D., Dorvillius, M., Gourgou, S., Martineau, P., Robert, B., Pugnière, M., Delard, R., Ychou, M., Dubois, J.B. & Pèlegrin, A. (2003a). Enhancement of radiation therapy by tumor necrosis factor alpha in human colon cancer using a bispecific antibody. *Int J Radiat Oncol Biol Phys*, **55**, 1363-73.

Azria, D., Larbouret, C., Martineau, P., Robert, B., Aillères, N., Ychou, M., Dubois, J.B. & Pèlegrin, A. (2003b). A Bispecific antibody against tumor necrosis factor alpha and carcinoembryonic antigen (CEA) to enhance radiation therapy in CEA-expressing digestive tumors. *Int J Radiat Oncol Biol Phys, In Press*.

Azria, D., Labouret, C., Garambois, V., Kramar, A., Martineau, P., Robert B., Aillères, N., Ychou, M., Dubois, J., & Pelegrin, A., (2004). Potentiation of ionising radiation by targeting tumour necrosis factor alpha using a biospecific antibody in human pancreatic cancer: *Brit J Cancer*, In press

Balaban, N., Moni, J., Shannon, M., Dang, L., Murphy, E. & Goldkorn, T. (1996). The effect of ionizing radiation on signal transduction: antibodies to EGF receptor sensitize A431 cells to radiation. *Biochim Biophys Acta*, **1314**, 147-56.

Barker, F.G., 2nd, Simmons, M.L., Chang, S.M., Prados, M.D., Larson, D.A., Sneed, P.K., Wara, W.M., Berger, M.S., Chen, P., Israel, M.A. & Aldape, K.D. (2001). EGFR overexpression and radiation response in glioblastoma multiforme. *Int J Radiat Oncol Biol Phys*, **51**, 410-8.

Baselga, J. (2001). The EGFR as a target for anticancer therapy--focus on cetuximab. *Eur J Cancer*, **37 Suppl 4**, S16-22.

Baselga, J. & Albanell, J. (2001). Mechanism of action of anti-HER2 monoclonal antibodies. *Ann Oncol*, **12**, S35-41.

Baselga, J., Norton, L., Albanell, J., Kim, Y.M. & Mendelsohn, J. (1998). Recombinant humanized anti-HER2 antibody (Herceptin) enhances the antitumor activity of paclitaxel and doxorubicin against HER2/neu overexpressing human breast cancer xenografts. *Cancer Res*, **58**, 2825-31.

Baselga, J., Pfister, D., Cooper, M.R., Cohen, R., Burtness, B., Bos, M., D'Andrea, G., Seidman, A., Norton, L., Gunnett, K., Falcey, J., Anderson, V., Waksal, H. & Mendelsohn, J. (2000). Phase I studies of anti-epidermal growth factor receptor chimeric antibody C225 alone and in combination with cisplatin. *J Clin Oncol*, **18**, 904-14.

Baselga, J., Tripathy, D., Mendelsohn, J., Baughman, S., Benz, C.C., Dantis, L., Sklarin, N.T., Seidman, A.D., Hudis, C.A., Moore, J., Rosen, P.P., Twaddell, T., Henderson, I.C. & Norton, L. (1996). Phase II study of weekly intravenous recombinant humanized anti-p185HER2 monoclonal antibody in patients with HER2/neu-overexpressing metastatic breast cancer. *J Clin Oncol*, **14**, 737-44.

Berger, M.S., Locher, G.W., Saurer, S., Gullick, W.J., Waterfield, M.D., Groner, B. & Hynes, N.E. (1988). Correlation of c-erbB-2 gene amplification and protein expression in human breast carcinoma with nodal status and nuclear grading. *Cancer Res*, **48**, 1238-43.

Beutler, B. & Cerami, A. (1988). The history, properties, and biological effects of cachectin. *Biochemistry*, **27**, 7575-82.

Bianco, C., Bianco, R., Tortora, G., Damiano, V., Guerrieri, P., Montemaggi, P., Mendelsohn, J., De Placido, S., Bianco, A.R. & Ciardiello, F. (2000). Antitumor activity of combined treatment of human cancer cells with ionizing radiation and anti-epidermal growth factor receptor monoclonal antibody C225 plus type I protein kinase A antisense oligonucleotide. *Clin Cancer Res*, **6**, 4343-50.

Bishop, J.M. (1991). Molecular themes in oncogenesis. *Cell*, **64**, 235-48.

Bonner, J.A., Ezekiel, M.P., Robert, F., Meredith, R.F., Spencer, S.A. & Waksal, H.W. (2000a). Continued response following treatment with IMC-C225, an EGFr MoAb, combined with RT in advanced head and neck malignancies. In *Proc ASCO*, Vol. 19 (5F). pp. 4a.

Bonner, J.A., Raisch, K.P., Trummell, H.Q., Robert, F., Meredith, R.F., Spencer, S.A., Buchsbaum, D.J., Saleh, M.N., Stackhouse, M.A., LoBuglio, A.F., Peters, G.E., Carroll, W.R. & Waksal, H.W. (2000b). Enhanced apoptosis with combination C225/radiation treatment serves as the impetus for clinical investigation in head and neck cancers. *J Clin Oncol*, **18**, 47S-53S.

Buchsbaum, D.J., Bonner, J.A., Grizzle, W.E., Stackhouse, M.A., Carpenter, M., Hicklin, D.J., Bohlen, P. & Raisch, K.P. (2002). Treatment of pancreatic cancer xenografts with Erbitux (IMC-C225) anti- EGFR antibody, gemcitabine, and radiation. *Int J Radiat Oncol Biol Phys*, **54**, 1180-93.

Carpenter, G. & Cohen, S. (1990). Epidermal growth factor. *J Biol Chem*, **265**, 7709-12.

Carswell, E.A., Old, L.J., Kassel, R.L., Green, S., Fiore, N. & Williamson, B. (1975). An endotoxin-induced serum factor that causes necrosis of tumors. *Proc Natl Acad Sci U S A*, **72**, 3666-70.

Carter, P., Presta, L., Gorman, C.M., Ridgway, J.B., Henner, D., Wong, W.L., Rowland, A.M., Kotts, C., Carver, M.E. & Shepard, H.M. (1992). Humanization of an anti-p185HER2 antibody for human cancer therapy. *Proc Natl Acad Sci U S A*, **89**, 4285-9.

Carter, S., Auer, K.L., Reardon, D.B., Birrer, M., Fisher, P.B., Valerie, K., Schmidt-Ullrich, R., Mikkelsen, R. & Dent, P. (1998). Inhibition of the mitogen activated protein (MAP) kinase cascade potentiates cell killing by low dose ionizing radiation in A431 human squamous carcinoma cells. *Oncogene*, **16**, 2787-96.

Chen, R.H., Su, Y.H., Chuang, R.L. & Chang, T.Y. (1998). Suppression of transforming growth factor-beta-induced apoptosis through a phosphatidylinositol 3-kinase/Akt-dependent pathway. *Oncogene*, **17**, 1959-68.

Chmura, S.J., Mauceri, H.J., Advani, S., Heimann, R., Beckett, M.A., Nodzenski, E., Quintans, J., Kufe, D.W. & Weichselbaum, R.R. (1997). Decreasing the apoptotic threshold of tumor cells through protein kinase C inhibition and sphingomyelinase activation increases tumor killing by ionizing radiation. *Cancer Res*, **57**, 4340-7.

Ciardiello, F. & Tortora, G. (2001). A novel approach in the treatment of cancer: targeting the epidermal growth factor receptor. *Clin Cancer Res*, **7**, 2958-70.

Clynes, R.A., Towers, T.L., Presta, L.G. & Ravetch, J.V. (2000). Inhibitory Fc receptors modulate in vivo cytoxicity against tumor targets. *Nat Med*, **6**, 443-6.

Cobleigh, M.A., Vogel, C.L., Tripathy, D., Robert, N.J., Scholl, S., Fehrenbacher, L., Wolter, J.M., Paton, V., Shak, S., Lieberman, G. & Slamon, D.J. (1999). Multinational study of the efficacy and safety of humanized anti-HER2 monoclonal antibody in women who have HER2-overexpressing metastatic breast cancer that has progressed after chemotherapy for metastatic disease. *J Clin Oncol*, **17**, 2639-48.

David, M., Wong, L., Flavell, R., Thompson, S.A., Wells, A., Larner, A.C. & Johnson, G.R. (1996). STAT activation by epidermal growth factor (EGF) and amphiregulin. Requirement for the EGF receptor kinase but not for tyrosine phosphorylation sites or JAK1. *J Biol Chem*, **271**, 9185-8.

Dent, P., Reardon, D.B., Morrison, D.K. & Sturgill, T.W. (1995). Regulation of Raf-1 and Raf-1 mutants by Ras-dependent and Ras-independent mechanisms in vitro. *Mol Cell Biol*, **15**, 4125-35.

Dent, P., Reardon, D.B., Park, J.S., Bowers, G., Logsdon, C., Valerie, K. & Schmidt-Ullrich, R. (1999). Radiation-induced release of transforming growth factor alpha activates the epidermal growth factor receptor and mitogen-activated protein kinase pathway in carcinoma cells, leading to increased proliferation and protection from radiation-induced cell death. *Mol Biol Cell*, **10**, 2493-506.

Di Fiore, P.P., Pierce, J.H., Kraus, M.H., Segatto, O., King, C.R. & Aaronson, S.A. (1987). erbB-2 is a potent oncogene when overexpressed in NIH/3T3 cells. *Science*, **237**, 178-82.

Dougall, W.C., Qian, X., Peterson, N.C., Miller, M.J., Samanta, A. & Greene, M.I. (1994). The neu-oncogene: signal transduction pathways, transformation mechanisms and evolving therapies. *Oncogene*, **9**, 2109-23.

Franke, T.F., Kaplan, D.R. & Cantley, L.C. (1997). PI3K: downstream AKTion blocks apoptosis. *Cell*, **88**, 435-7.

Ghosh, S., Strum, J.C., Sciorra, V.A., Daniel, L. & Bell, R.M. (1996). Raf-1 kinase possesses distinct binding domains for phosphatidylserine and phosphatidic acid. Phosphatidic acid regulates the translocation of Raf-1 in 12-O-tetradecanoylphorbol-13-acetate-stimulated Madin-Darby canine kidney cells. *J Biol Chem*, **271**, 8472-80.

Goldkorn, T., Balaban, N., Shannon, M. & Matsukuma, K. (1997). EGF receptor phosphorylation is affected by ionizing radiation. *Biochim Biophys Acta*, **1358**, 289-99.

Goldstein, N.I., Prewett, M., Zuklys, K., Rockwell, P. & Mendelsohn, J. (1995). Biological efficacy of a chimeric antibody to the epidermal growth factor receptor in a human tumor xenograft model. *Clin Cancer Res*, **1**, 1311-8.

Grandis, J.R., Drenning, S.D., Zeng, Q., Watkins, S.C., Melhem, M.F., Endo, S., Johnson, D.E., Huang, L., He, Y. & Kim, J.D. (2000). Constitutive activation of Stat3 signaling abrogates apoptosis in squamous cell carcinogenesis in vivo. *Proc Natl Acad Sci U S A*, **97**, 4227-32.

Gridley, D.S., Archambeau, J.O., Andres, M.A., Mao, X.W., Wright, K. & Slater, J.M. (1997). Tumor necrosis factor-alpha enhances antitumor effects of radiation against glioma xenografts. *Oncol Res*, **9**, 217-27.

Gridley, D.S., Hammond, S.N. & Liwnicz, B.H. (1994). Tumor necrosis factor-alpha augments radiation effects against human colon tumor xenografts. *Anticancer Res*, **14**, 1107-12.

Gupta, A.K., McKenna, W.G., Weber, C.N., Feldman, M.D., Goldsmith, J.D., Mick, R., Machtay, M., Rosenthal, D.I., Bakanauskas, V.J., Cerniglia, G.J., Bernhard, E.J., Weber, R.S. & Muschel, R.J. (2002). Local recurrence in head and neck cancer: relationship to radiation resistance and signal transduction. *Clin Cancer Res*, **8**, 885-92.

Guy, P.M., Platko, J.V., Cantley, L.C., Cerione, R.A. & Carraway, K.L., 3rd. (1994). Insect cell-expressed p180erbB3 possesses an impaired tyrosine kinase activity. *Proc Natl Acad Sci U S A*, **91**, 8132-6.

Haimovitz-Friedman, A. (1998). Radiation-induced signal transduction and stress response. *Radiat Res*, **150**, S102-8.

Hallahan, D.E., Beckett, M.A., Kufe, D. & Weichselbaum, R.R. (1990). The interaction between recombinant human tumor necrosis factor and radiation in 13 human tumor cell lines. *Int J Radiat Oncol Biol Phys*, **19**, 69-74.

Hambek, M., Solbach, C., Schnuerch, H.G., Roller, M., Stegmueller, M., Sterner-Kock, A., Kiefer, J. & Knecht, R. (2001). Tumor necrosis factor alpha sensitizes low epidermal growth factor receptor (EGFR)-expressing carcinomas for anti-EGFR therapy. *Cancer Res*, **61**, 1045-9.

Helson, L., Helson, C. & Green, S. (1979). Effects of murine tumor necrosis factor on heterotransplanted human tumors. *Exp Cell Biol*, **47**, 53-60.

Huang, S.M., Bock, J.M. & Harari, P.M. (1999). Epidermal growth factor receptor blockade with C225 modulates proliferation, apoptosis, and radiosensitivity in squamous cell carcinomas of the head and neck. *Cancer Res*, **59**, 1935-40.

Huang, S.M. & Harari, P.M. (1999). Epidermal growth factor receptor inhibition in cancer therapy: biology, rationale and preliminary clinical results. *Invest New Drugs*, **17**, 259-69.

Huang, S.M. & Harari, P.M. (2000). Modulation of radiation response after epidermal growth factor receptor blockade in squamous cell carcinomas: inhibition of damage repair, cell cycle kinetics, and tumor angiogenesis. *Clin Cancer Res*, **6**, 2166-74.

Hudziak, R.M., Lewis, G.D., Winget, M., Fendly, B.M., Shepard, H.M. & Ullrich, A. (1989). p185HER2 monoclonal antibody has antiproliferative effects in vitro and sensitizes human breast tumor cells to tumor necrosis factor. *Mol Cell Biol*, **9**, 1165-72.

Hudziak, R.M., Schlessinger, J. & Ullrich, A. (1987). Increased expression of the putative growth factor receptor p185HER2 causes transformation and tumorigenesis of NIH 3T3 cells. *Proc Natl Acad Sci U S A*, **84**, 7159-63.

Hynes, N.E. & Stern, D.F. (1994). The biology of erbB-2/neu/HER-2 and its role in cancer. *Biochim Biophys Acta*, **1198**, 165-84.

Ignatoski, K.M., Lapointe, A.J., Radany, E.H. & Ethier, S.P. (1999). erbB-2 overexpression in human mammary epithelial cells confers growth factor independence. *Endocrinology*, **140**, 3615-22.

Izumi, Y., Xu, L., di Tomaso, E., Fukumura, D. & Jain, R.K. (2002). Tumour biology: Herceptin acts as an anti-angiogenic cocktail. *Nature*, **416**, 279-80.

Janes, P.W., Daly, R.J., deFazio, A. & Sutherland, R.L. (1994). Activation of the Ras signalling pathway in human breast cancer cells overexpressing erbB-2. *Oncogene*, **9**, 3601-8.

Jurianz, K., Maslak, S., Garcia-Schuler, H., Fishelson, Z. & Kirschfink, M. (1999). Neutralization of complement regulatory proteins augments lysis of breast carcinoma cells targeted with rhumAb anti-HER2. *Immunopharmacology*, **42**, 209-18.

Kavanagh, B.D., Dent, P., Schmidt-Ullrich, R.K., Chen, P. & Mikkelsen, R.B. (1998). Calcium-dependent stimulation of mitogen-activated protein kinase activity in A431 cells by low doses of ionizing radiation. *Radiat Res*, **149**, 579-87.

Klapper, L.N., Vaisman, N., Hurwitz, E., Pinkas-Kramarski, R., Yarden, Y. & Sela, M. (1997). A subclass of tumor-inhibitory monoclonal antibodies to ErbB-2/HER2 blocks crosstalk with growth factor receptors. *Oncogene*, **14**, 2099-109.

Lane, H.A., Motoyama, A.B., Beuvink, I. & Hynes, N.E. (2001). Modulation of p27/Cdk2 complex formation through 4D5-mediated inhibition of HER2 receptor signaling. *Ann Oncol*, **12**, S21-2.

Lin, J.T., Wu, M.S., Shun, C.T., Lee, W.J., Sheu, J.C. & Wang, T.H. (1995). Occurrence of microsatellite instability in gastric carcinoma is associated with enhanced expression of erbB-2 oncoprotein. *Cancer Res*, **55**, 1428-30.

Marais, R., Light, Y., Paterson, H.F. & Marshall, C.J. (1995). Ras recruits Raf-1 to the plasma membrane for activation by tyrosine phosphorylation. *Embo J*, **14**, 3136-45.

Milas, L., Mason, K., Hunter, N., Petersen, S., Yamakawa, M., Ang, K., Mendelsohn, J. & Fan, Z. (2000). In vivo enhancement of tumor radioresponse by C225 antiepidermal growth factor receptor antibody. *Clin Cancer Res*, **6**, 701-8.

Moghal, N. & Sternberg, P.W. (1999). Multiple positive and negative regulators of signaling by the EGF-receptor. *Curr Opin Cell Biol*, **11**, 190-6.

Moscatello, D.K., Holgado-Madruga, M., Emlet, D.R., Montgomery, R.B. & Wong, A.J. (1998). Constitutive activation of phosphatidylinositol 3-kinase by a naturally occurring mutant epidermal growth factor receptor. *J Biol Chem*, **273**, 200-6.

Naramura, M., Gillies, S.D., Mendelsohn, J., Reisfeld, R.A. & Mueller, B.M. (1993). Therapeutic potential of chimeric and murine anti-(epidermal growth factor receptor) antibodies in a metastasis model for human melanoma. *Cancer Immunol Immunother*, **37**, 343-9.

Nasu, S., Ang, K.K., Fan, Z. & Milas, L. (2001). C225 antiepidermal growth factor receptor antibody enhances tumor radiocurability. *Int J Radiat Oncol Biol Phys*, **51**, 474-7.

Nicholson, R.I., Gee, J.M. & Harper, M.E. (2001). EGFR and cancer prognosis. *Eur J Cancer*, **37 Suppl 4**, S9-15.

Nishiguchi, I., Willingham, V. & Milas, L. (1990). Tumor necrosis factor as an adjunct to fractionated radiotherapy in the treatment of murine tumors. *Int J Radiat Oncol Biol Phys*, **18**, 555-8.

Old, L.J. (1988). Tumor necrosis factor. *Sci Am*, **258**, 59-60, 69-75.

O'Rourke, D.M., Kao, G.D., Singh, N., Park, B.W., Muschel, R.J., Wu, C.J. & Greene, M.I. (1998). Conversion of a radioresistant phenotype to a more sensitive one by disabling erbB receptor signaling in human cancer cells. *Proc. Natl. Acad.Sci. USA*, **95**, 10842-10847.

Park, O.K., Schaefer, T.S. & Nathans, D. (1996). In vitro activation of Stat3 by epidermal growth factor receptor kinase. *Proc Natl Acad Sci U S A*, **93**, 13704-8.

Pegram, M.D., Lipton, A., Hayes, D.F., Weber, B.L., Baselga, J.M., Tripathy, D., Baly, D., Baughman, S.A., Twaddell, T., Glaspy, J.A. & Slamon, D.J. (1998). Phase II study of receptor-enhanced chemosensitivity using recombinant humanized anti-p185HER2/neu monoclonal antibody plus cisplatin in patients with HER2/neu-overexpressing metastatic breast cancer refractory to chemotherapy treatment. *J Clin Oncol*, **16**, 2659-71.

Peng, D., Fan, Z., Lu, Y., DeBlasio, T., Scher, H. & Mendelsohn, J. (1996). Anti-epidermal growth factor receptor monoclonal antibody 225 up-regulates p27KIP1 and induces G1 arrest in prostatic cancer cell line DU145. *Cancer Res*, **56**, 3666-9.

Perrotte, P., Matsumoto, T., Inoue, K., Kuniyasu, H., Eve, B.Y., Hicklin, D.J., Radinsky, R. & Dinney, C.P. (1999). Anti-epidermal growth factor receptor antibody C225 inhibits angiogenesis in human transitional cell carcinoma growing orthotopically in nude mice. *Clin Cancer Res*, **5**, 257-65.

Perry, J.E., Grossmann, M.E. & Tindall, D.J. (1998). Epidermal growth factor induces cyclin D1 in a human prostate cancer cell line. *Prostate*, **35**, 117-24.

Petit, A.M., Rak, J., Hung, M.C., Rockwell, P., Goldstein, N., Fendly, B. & Kerbel, R.S. (1997). Neutralizing antibodies against epidermal growth factor and ErbB-2/neu receptor tyrosine kinases down-regulate vascular endothelial growth factor production by tumor cells in vitro and in vivo: angiogenic implications for signal transduction therapy of solid tumors. *Am J Pathol*, **151**, 1523-30.

Pietras, R.J., Poen, J.C., Gallardo, D., Wongvipat, P.N., Lee, H.J. & Slamon, D.J. (1999). Monoclonal antibody to HER-2/neureceptor modulates repair of radiation-induced DNA damage and enhances radiosensitivity of human breast cancer cells overexpressing this oncogene. *Cancer Res*, **59**, 1347-55.

Prewett, M., Rothman, M., Waksal, H., Feldman, M., Bander, N.H. & Hicklin, D.J. (1998). Mouse-human chimeric anti-epidermal growth factor receptor antibody C225 inhibits the growth of human renal cell carcinoma xenografts in nude mice. *Clin Cancer Res*, **4**, 2957-66.

Radinsky, R., Risin, Fan, Dong, Bielenberg, Bucana & Fidler. (1995). Level and function of epidermal growth factor receptor predict the metastatic potential of human colon carcinoma cells. *Clin Cancer Res*, **1**, 19-31.

Ram, T.G. & Ethier, S.P. (1996). Phosphatidylinositol 3-kinase recruitment by p185erbB-2 and erbB-3 is potently induced by neu differentiation factor/heregulin during mitogenesis and is constitutively elevated in growth factor-independent breast carcinoma cells with c-erbB-2 gene amplification. *Cell Growth Differ*, **7**, 551-61.

Robert, B., Mach, J.P., Mani, J.C., Ychou, M., Folli, S., Artus, J.C. & Pelegrin, A. (1996). Cytokine targeting in tumors using a bispecific antibody directed against carcinoembryonic antigen and tumor necrosis factor alpha. *Cancer Res*, **56**, 4758-65.

Ruegg, C., Yilmaz, A., Bieler, G., Bamat, J., Chaubert, P. & Lejeune, F.J. (1998). Evidence for the involvement of endothelial cell integrin alphaVbeta3 in the disruption of the tumor vasculature induced by TNF and IFN-gamma. *Nat Med*, **4**, 408-14.

Saleh, M.N., Raisch, K.P., Stackhouse, M.A., Grizzle, W.E., Bonner, J.A., Mayo, M.S., Kim, H.G., Meredith, R.F., Wheeler, R.H. & Buchsbaum, D.J. (1999). Combined modality therapy of A431 human epidermoid cancer using anti-EGFr antibody C225 and radiation. *Cancer Biother Radiopharm*, **14**, 451-63.

Santana, P., Pena, L.A., Haimovitz-Friedman, A., Martin, S., Green, D., McLoughlin, M., Cordon-Cardo, C., Schuchman, E.H., Fuks, Z. & Kolesnick, R. (1996). Acid sphingomyelinase-deficient human lymphoblasts and mice are defective in radiation-induced apoptosis. *Cell*, **86**, 189-99.

Schmidt, M., McWatters, A., White, R.A., Groner, B., Wels, W., Fan, Z. & Bast, R.C., Jr. (2001). Synergistic interaction between an anti-p185HER-2 pseudomonas exotoxin fusion protein [scFv(FRP5)-ETA] and ionizing radiation for inhibiting growth of ovarian cancer cells that overexpress HER-2. *Gynecol Oncol*, **80**, 145-55.

Schmidt-Ullrich, R.K., Dent, P., Grant, S., Mikkelsen, R.B. & Valerie, K. (2000). Signal transduction and cellular radiation responses. *Radiat Res*, **153**, 245-57.

Schmidt-Ullrich, R.K., Mikkelsen, R.B., Dent, P., Todd, D.G., Valerie, K., Kavanagh, B.D., Contessa, J.N., Rorrer, W.K. & Chen, P.B. (1997). Radiation-induced proliferation of the human A431 squamous carcinoma cells is dependent on EGFR tyrosine phosphorylation. *Oncogene*, **15**, 1191-7.

Schnurch, H.G., Stegmuller, M., Vering, A., Beckmann, M.W. & Bender, H.G. (1994). Growth inhibition of xenotransplanted human carcinomas by a monoclonal antibody directed against the epidermal growth factor receptor. *Eur J Cancer*, **4**, 491-6.

Sersa, G., Willingham, V. & Milas, L. (1988). Anti-tumor effects of tumor necrosis factor alone or combined with radiotherapy. *Int J Cancer*, **42**, 129-34.

Shak, S. (1999). Overview of the trastuzumab (Herceptin) anti-HER2 monoclonal antibody clinical program in HER2-overexpressing metastatic breast cancer. Herceptin Multinational Investigator Study Group. *Semin Oncol*, **26**, 71-7.

Slamon, D.J., Leyland-Jones, B., Shak, S., Fuchs, H., Paton, V., Bajamonde, A., Fleming, T., Eiermann, W., Wolter, J., Pegram, M., Baselga, J. & Norton, L. (2001). Use of chemotherapy plus a monoclonal antibody against HER2 for metastatic breast cancer that overexpresses HER2. *N Engl J Med*, **344**, 783-92.

Slichenmyer, W.J. & Fry, D.W. (2001). Anticancer therapy targeting the erbB family of receptor tyrosine kinases. *Semin Oncol*, **28**, 67-79.

Sliwkowski, M.X., Lofgren, J.A., Lewis, G.D., Hotaling, T.E., Fendly, B.M. & Fox, J.A. (1999). Nonclinical studies addressing the mechanism of action of trastuzumab (Herceptin). *Semin Oncol*, **26**, 60-70.

Stackhouse, M.A., Buchsbaum, D.J., Grizzle, W.E., Bright, S.J., Olsen, C.C., Kancharla, S., Mayo, M.S. & Curiel, D.T. (1998). Radiosensitization mediated by a transfected anti-erbB-2 single-chain antibody in vitro and in vivo. *Int J Radiat Oncol Biol Phys*, **42**, 817-22.

Sugarman, B.J., Aggarwal, B.B., Hass, P.E., Figari, I.S., Palladino, M.A., Jr. & Shepard, H.M. (1985). Recombinant human tumor necrosis factor-alpha: effects on proliferation of normal and transformed cells in vitro. *Science*, **230**, 943-5.

Teramoto, T., Onda, M., Tokunaga, A. & Asano, G. (1996). Inhibitory effect of anti-epidermal growth factor receptor antibody on a human gastric cancer. *Cancer*, **77**, 1639-45.

Tokuda, Y., Ohnishi, Y., Shimamura, K., Iwasawa, M., Yoshimura, M., Ueyama, Y., Tamaoki, N., Tajima, T. & Mitomi, T. (1996). In vitro and in vivo anti-tumour effects of a humanised monoclonal antibody against c-erbB-2 product. *Br J Cancer*, **73**, 1362-5.

Tombes, R.M., Auer, K.L., Mikkelsen, R., Valerie, K., Wymann, M.P., Marshall, C.J., McMahon, M. & Dent, P. (1998). The mitogen-activated protein (MAP) kinase cascade can either stimulate or inhibit DNA synthesis in primary cultures of rat hepatocytes depending upon whether its activation is acute/phasic or chronic. *Biochem J*, **330** (**Pt 3)**, 1451-60.

Tse, C., Brault, D. & Etienne, J. (1997). [Current aspects of the evaluation of ERBB2 activation in breast cancer. Therapeutic perspectives]. *Ann Biol Clin (Paris)*, **55**, 545-54.

Ullrich, A. & Schlessinger, J. (1990). Signal transduction by receptors with tyrosine kinase activity. *Cell*, **61**, 203-12.

Uno, M., Otsuki, T., Kurebayashi, J., Sakaguchi, H., Isozaki, Y., Ueki, A., Yata, K., Fujii, T., Hiratsuka, J., Akisada, T., Harada, T. & Imajo, Y. (2001). Anti-HER2-antibody enhances irradiation-induced growth inhibition in head and neck carcinoma. *Int J Cancer*, **94**, 474-9.

van der Geer, P., Hunter, T. & Lindberg, R.A. (1994). Receptor protein-tyrosine kinases and their signal transduction pathways. *Annu Rev Cell Biol*, **10**, 251-337.

Voldborg, B.R., Damstrup, L., Spang-Thomsen, M. & Poulsen, H.S. (1997). Epidermal growth factor receptor (EGFR) and EGFR mutations, function and possible role in clinical trials. *Ann Oncol*, **8**, 1197-206.

Warenius, H.M., Jones, M.D. & Thompson, C.C. (1996). Exit from G2 phase after 2 Gy gamma irradiation is faster in radiosensitive human cells with high expression of the RAF1 proto-oncogene. *Radiat Res*, **146**, 485-93.

Wollman, R., Yahalom, J., Maxy, R., Pinto, J. & Fuks, Z. (1994). Effect of epidermal growth factor on the growth and radiation sensitivity of human breast cancer cells in vitro. *Int J Radiat Oncol Biol Phys*, **30**, 91-8.

Wu, X., Fan, Z., Masui, H., Rosen, N. & Mendelsohn, J. (1995). Apoptosis induced by an anti-epidermal growth factor receptor monoclonal antibody in a human colorectal carcinoma cell line and its delay by insulin. *J Clin Invest*, **95**, 1897-905.

Wu, X., Rubin, M., Fan, Z., DeBlasio, T., Soos, T., Koff, A. & Mendelsohn, J. (1996). Involvement of p27KIP1 in G1 arrest mediated by an anti-epidermal growth factor receptor monoclonal antibody. *Oncogene*, **12**, 1397-403.

Xia, Z., Dickens, M., Raingeaud, J., Davis, R.J. & Greenberg, M.E. (1995). Opposing effects of ERK and JNK-p38 MAP kinases on apoptosis. *Science*, **270**, 1326-31.

Yarden, Y. (2001). The EGFR family and its ligands in human cancer. signalling mechanisms and therapeutic opportunities. *Eur J Cancer*, **37 Suppl 4**, S3-8.

Yarden, Y. & Ullrich, A. (1988). Growth factor receptor tyrosine kinases. *Annu Rev Biochem*, **57**, 443-78.

Zolfaghari, A. & Djakiew, D. (1996). Inhibition of chemomigration of a human prostatic carcinoma cell (TSU-pr1) line by inhibition of epidermal growth factor receptor function. *Prostate*, **28**, 232-8.

zum Buschenfelde, C.M., Hermann, C., Schmidt, B., Peschel, C. & Bernhard, H. (2002). Antihuman Epidermal Growth Factor Receptor 2 (HER2) Monoclonal Antibody Trastuzumab Enhances Cytolytic Activity of Class I-restricted HER2-specific T Lymphocytes Against HER2-overexpressing Tumor Cells. *Cancer Res*, **62**, 2244-7.

Chapter 7

ANTIBODIES, A POTENT TOOL TO TARGET GENES INTO DESIGNATED CELLS AND TISSUES

Francois Hirsch[*], Olivier Deas[*$], Gabrielle Carvalho[*], Antoine Dürrbach[*], Dominique Thierry[#] and Alain Chapel[#]

[*]Inserm unit 542, Paris-Sud University, GDR 2352 "immunotargeting of tumors" and [$]Targa Therapies, Villejuif; [#]Institute of Radioprotection and Nuclear Safety, IRSN/DPHD/SARAM, Fontenay-aux-Roses, France

1. INTRODUCTION

After a period of euphoria following the report on the first *ex vivo* production of monoclonal antibodies (Kohler, 1975), the new "magic bullets" as they were qualified by the press, however did not keep theirs promise. Indeed, apart OKT3 a mouse mAb directed against the T lymphocyte CD3 molecule, the first to get US and European approvals in the prevention of organ rejection in 1986, several trials conducted with other mAbs did not show significant results. These poor effects were mainly due to generation of anti-murine Abs by the patients, hindering the efficacy of the treatment. Moreover, rodent IgG Abs injected to patients have half-life of less than 20 hrs compared to several days for human Igs.

Nevertheless, mAbs slowly but surely modified medicine. For instance, diagnostic methods were markedly improved by the introduction of radio- or fluorescent-labeled mAbs permitting the detection of normal or pathologic cell subpopulations *in vitro* but also *in vivo*. Mabs also modified production processes used to purify proteins. As such, the design of mAbs-coated beads capable of immunopurifying large amounts of molecules greatly expanded the production of high quality human-derived proteins (seric proteins, hormones...).

Table 7.1. Monoclonal antibodies approved in the EU and in the USA.

Trade name	Targeted antigen	Indication	Marketing
CAMPATH	CD52 on normal and malign B- and T-lymphocytes	Therapy of CLL	EU, USA
CEA-SCAN	CEA	*In vivo*-diagnosis of colon-or rectum carcinoma	EU
HERCEPTIN	Extracellular domain of the human Epidermal Growth Factor 2 (HER 2)	Treatment of metastatic breast cancer	EU, USA
HUMASPECT	Tumor-associated antigen-complex (cytokeratin-polypeptide MW 35-43)	*In vivo* -diagnosis of colon-or rectum carcinoma	EU
LEUKOSCAN	Surface glycoprotein NCA90 on granulocytes and CEA	*In vivo* -diagnosis of osteomyelitis	EU
MYELOTARG	CD33	Acute myelogenous leukaemia	USA
ORTHOCLONE OKT3	CD3 on T-lymphocytes	Therapy of acute steroid resistant rejection episodes in allogenic kidney, heart and liver transplantation	EU, USA
MABTHERA	CD20 on pre-B-and mature B-lymphocytes	Treatment of B-cell-non-Hodgkin-Lymphoma (in combination with CHOP chemotherapy) Treatment of chemoresistant follicular lymphoma	EU, USA
REMICADE	Soluble and transmembrane TNFα	Rheumatoid Arthritis, Crohn's disease	EU, USA
REOPRO	GPIIb/IIIa ($\alpha_{IIb}\beta_3$)-receptor of thrombocytes and Vitronectin ($\alpha_v\beta_3$) receptor of thrombocytes and epithelial cells	Inhibitor of thrombocyte aggregation	EU, USA
SIMULECT	Alpha-subunit of IL2-receptor on activated T-lymphocytes (CD25)	Prophylaxis of acute rejection episodes in allogenic de *novo* kidney transplantation	EU, USA
SYNARGIS	A-Epitop of the Fusion protein of RSV	Prevention of Respiratory Syncitial Virus disease in infants at risk	EU, USA
ZENAPAX	Alpha-subunit of IL2-receptor on activated T-Lymphocytes (CD25)	Prophylaxis of acute rejection episodes in allogenic de *novo* kidney transplantation	EU, USA

Thanks to the development of genetic engineering, chimeric and humanized mAbs were developed in the nineteen's, leading to an increase in approval of mAbs intended for therapeutic use by the EMEA (European medical agency for the evaluation of medical products) and the USA-FDA (Federal Drug Agency) (**Table 7.1**).

Moreover, hundreds are in clinical trials in fields that no one could anticipate 30 years ago, cancer and transplant rejection for the majority but also autoimmune diseases, asthma, cardiology and infectious diseases. In parallel, an expanding field mainly in cancer therapy is the use of mAbs as carrier of cytotoxic agents inside the tumors. Various molecules were tested, as illustrated in other chapters of this book: radionucleides, toxins, prodrug and more recently chimiotherapeutic drugs.

Given the targeting properties of mAbs, some groups like ours proposed to use them to convey DNA molecules encoding therapeutic molecules into designated cells. In this chapter, we will provide an overview on the various approaches chosen to target genes. Through two different models, we will also try to demonstrate that indeed mAbs should be of great interest for gene transfer. As a cautionary note, this survey does not pretend to be exhaustive, but rather to appeal to the reader's curiosity.

2.   ANTIBODY AS GENE CARRIER

The design of strategies allowing the specific targeting of genes, that is their expression in a limited subset of cells, is now the major issue of gene therapy. To date, only very few procedures permit cell- or tissue-specific targeting *in vivo*. For instance, 80% of the almost 600 clinical trials in cancer gene therapy are based on direct intratumoral administration of recombinant vectors and/or on *ex vivo* cell manipulations (Weichselbaum, 1997). Although viral vectors allow efficient and long-term gene expression, they generally don't permit gene delivery into designated target cells. Thus, there has been an intense interest on methods that would allow specific gene delivery and many laboratories are now dealing with this exciting challenge.

As illustrated in **Figure 7.1**, the ideal vector should be able (i) to target the appropriate cells, (ii) to get into the cells, (iii) to escape the various traps present into cells, i.e. the endosomal pathway in which the vector can be retained and the cytosol rich in nucleases, (iv) to enter the nucleus where is located the transcription machinery.

Figure 7.1 The ideal vector should be able (1) to target the appropriate cells, (2) to enter into the cell nucleus, to permit gene transcription machinery (3), protein synthesis (4) and then protein secretion (5).

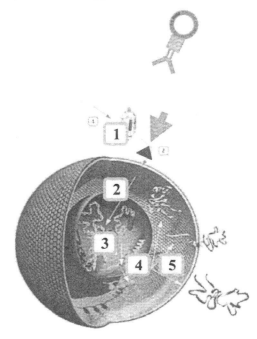

1) Targeting and entry of the vector
2) Nucleus entry
3) Transcription
4) Protein synthesis
5) Protein secretion

2.1   Design of a targeted vector

To allow cell targeting, attempts have been undertaken by several groups, using receptor-mediated gene transfer technologies. Numerous studies with transferrin as ligand have shown effective gene transfer delivery into various cell types (Wagner, 1990; Zenke, 1990; Schwarzenberger, 1996). Also asialo-orosomucoid was used to target asialoglycoproteins (Perales, 1994). However, most of the ligands tested so far are either broadly expressed (Wagner, 1990) or limited to one organ such as the liver (Perales, 1994).

Among the various approaches under investigation, the use of Abs to achieve tissue specific targeting constitutes a promising tool. Numerous mAbs recognizing defined targets, and with known tissue distribution are already in use in clinical trials and have been approved by international regulatory authorities, as reported above. In particular, several Abs are directed to cell specific Ags, such as the family of CD (cluster of differentiation) molecules specifically present on a large number of cells (for reference see http://www.ncbi.nlm.nih.gov/PROW/guide/45277084.htm), or the tumor-associated Ag (TAA) with a widely restricted expression (Roselli, 1996; Wang, 1999). These particular mAbs thus constitute some highly valuable tools.

As mentioned above, viruses represent the main category of vectors used in gene transfer with however a poor specificity. In order to improve this specificity some groups have designed targeted viruses.

Retroviruses the major gene-delivery vehicle, with high transduction efficiency, are able to containing DNA insert size up to 8 kb. The integration into host genome results in sustained expression of vector, but can bring mutagenic effects caused by random integration into the host genome. In a first attempt, viral targeting has been tested with divalent Abs linked by biotin-streptavidin conjugates, one directed to the retrovirus envelope protein, the other to a cell surface protein (Goud, 1988). Retroviruses may also be genetically modified to express a chimeric envelope containing single-chain variable fragments (scFv) with various Ag specificities (Pelegrin, 1998; Maurice, 2002).

Adenoviruses, also broadly utilized in gene therapy, have a high transduction efficiency, are capable of containing DNA inserts up to 8 kb, and infect both replicating and differentiated cells. Disadvantages of adenoviral vectors include a transient expression since the viral DNA does not integrate into the host, the expression of viral proteins following administration into the host. Moreover, adenoviral vectors are an extremely common human pathogen and *in vivo* delivery may be hampered by prior exacerbate host immune response to the virus, leading in some patients to severe inflammatory reactions. Targeting may be achieved by genetic engineering to suppress their native receptor interactions which are replaced by novel ligand genetically incorporated into virus coat proteins (Wickham, 2000).

A third class of virus, the adeno-associated virus (AAV) was designed to produce a gene therapy vector with site-specific integration and the ability to infect multiple cell types. This vector does offer some advantages over other vector systems which include the lack of initiating an immune response, their stability and ability to infect a variety of dividing and non-dividing cells. Unfortunately, they cannot incorporate genes larger than 5 kb. Targeting was approached using a bispecific F(ab'γ)2 Ab in which one arm recognizes a cell-specific ligand and the other the AAV capsid structure (Bartlett, 1999).

However, several questions remain before using these sophisticated constructs in clinics, regarding their pharmacokinetic properties after systemic administration, their real capacity to target cells without being trapped, their stability.

Non viral approaches may also be used through plasmid DNA conjugated to a ligand capable of binding to the surface of the targeted cells. The resulting conjugates retain their ability to specifically interact with cognate receptors on the cell surface. In this context, mAbs may represent a potent targeting tool. For instance, cationic liposomes complexed with DNA were extensively used *in vitro* and *in vivo* (reviewed in Templeton, 1997) lacking however target specificity due to lipid non-specific binding. Specificity was restored by the design of immunoliposomes upon conjugation of whole Ig, (Shi, 2000; Zhang, 2002) or Ig fragments, i.e. scFv (Xu, 2002) or Fab' (Mastrobattista, 2001).

Alternatively, mAbs may contribute to provide targeting ability to the so called lipoplexes obtained through the interactions of plasmid DNA and cationic polymers such as polylysine or polyethylenimines (Erbacher, 1999). This allowed *in vitro* gene delivery in neuroblastoma cell line (Erbacher, 1999) or in human peripheral mononuclear cells {O'Neill, 2001 #17}, or in human hematopoietic progenitor cell lines (Schwarzenberger, 1996).

The method we have developed is based on the production of hybrid molecules in which plasmid DNA is attached to mAbs recognizing surface Ags expressed on cells. Provided that the relevant Ag is internalized upon binding of the specific mAb, the plasmid can be expressed in a transitory fashion (**Figure 7.2**). Depending on the specificity of the mAb, thus reporter genes have been specifically targeted into various murine cells, B lymphocytes (anti-IgD Ab) or T lymphocytes (anti-CD3ε Ab), *in vitro* (Hirsch, 1993; Poncet, 1996), and *in vivo* (Poncet, 1996).

To further illustrate our model, we will report recent experiments aiming at transferring genes encoding therapeutic proteins into renal cancer cells or into hematopoietic progenitor cells.

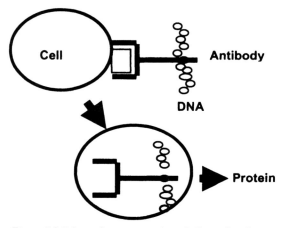

Figure 7.2 Schematic representation of Ab-mediated gene transfer

2.2 Antibody-mediated gene transfer into human renal tumor

Despite its relative low frequency, renal cancer due to its chemo- and radio-resistance, remains one of the most aggressive tumors without effective treatment, urging to find new therapeutic approaches (Mulders, 1997). In this context, our Ab-mediated gene transfer strategy was facilitated by the availability of the highly specific G250 mAb (Oosterwijk, 1986), already used in phase II trial (Oosterwijk, 1995) and capable of being internalized into renal cell carcinoma (RCC) upon binding to its Ag (Dürrbach, 1999). The human RCC utilized in these studies were derived from patients with primary tumors or metastases (Angevin, 1999).

In vitro, we first demonstrated that our vector construct carrying *β-galactosidase* applied to RCC was detected in 15 % of G250 RCC, while it was undetectable in untransfected RCC, nor was any ß-galactosidase expression detectable after incubation with the vector including an irrelevant mAb. In addition, no positive cells were detected when cells were incubated with the whole vector carrying an irrelevant plasmid DNA (Déas, 2002).

Moreover, efficient and specific gene delivery were achieved *in vivo*, in mice engrafted with tumor cells, G250 positive or G250 negative. When mice were intravenously injected with the vector containing cDNA encoding ß-galactosidase, the enzyme was detected in most of the G250 positive tumors, while it was not detected in the G250 negative tumors. In addition, expression of ß-galactosidase was not detected in liver, kidney, gut and spleen of all the injected animals (Déas, 2002).

These results led us to test the ability of our vectors in transferring a gene with therapeutic property in mice bearing RCC tumors. We choose the pro-apoptotic *bax* gene, one of the members of *bcl-2* family that promote apoptosis in modifying the balance between anti-apoptotic and pro-apoptotic proteins in cells (Knudson, 1997). When *bax* is over expressed in cells, they switched toward a pro-apoptotic status and died by direct action of bax or became sensitive or more sensitive to a second apoptotic signal induced by chemotherapies or radiotherapies (Tsuruta, 2001). *Bax* plays its tumor suppressor gene role with a direct dysfunctional effect on mitochondria which has a crucial role in cell death process. This dysfunctional effect on mitochondria induces the two apoptotic pathways identified today: one dependant of the clivage of specific cystein proteases named caspases (reviewed in Henkart, 1996), leading to the "classical apoptosis", and the other pathway, caspase-independent, resulting in necrosis phenotype. These two forms of death could promote immune system activation and elicit an antitumoral response, resulting in a bystander effect. In addition, *bax* was used *in vivo* to kill malignant cells in few models (Arafat, 2000; Tai, 1999).

We thus constructed a vector containing Bax encoding plasmid DNA conjugated to G250 mAb. As seen in **Figure 7.3**; *Bax* expression can induce RCC death *in vitro*, in a specific manner since only Bax encoding DNA conveyed with G250 mAb induced an important RCC loss. For *in vivo* therapeutic experiments, human renal carcinoma fragments (4 mm^3) were subcutaneously engrafted in irradiated nude mice. In the experiment shown in **Figure 7.4**, the vector including the cDNA *bax* linked to G250 mAb (**lane 1**) or the vector with the irrelevant anti-CD20 mAb (**lane 2**) or the cDNA *bax* only (**lane 3**) were intravenously injected once under anesthesia in the retro-orbital vein of animals bearing an established and vascularised tumor (2 weeks after engraftment) (**Figure 7.4** upper panel). As depicted on **Figure 7.4** lower panel, eight days following the injection, six out of nine mice treated with the vector carrying *bax* showed a significant decrease in the tumor growth (tumor size below the mean 495+/-38 mm^3) as compared to mice treated with the vector bearing an irrelevant mAb (one out of eight below 495+/-38 mm^3) or to the vector lacking mAb (none of nine below 495+/-38 mm^3). The effect of the entire vector on tumor growth was still noticeable up to day 18 following the injection. It is also of note that no toxicity was observed in the treated mice.

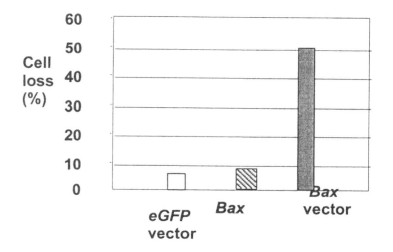

Figure 7.3 Effect of the in vitro transfer of Bax in G250 positive renal cell carcinoma

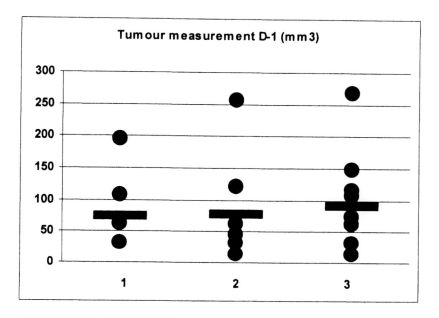

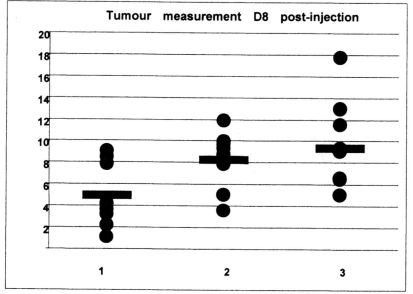

Figure 7.4 Effect of the in vivo transfer of bax gene into grafted G250 positive renal cell carcinoma

2.3   Antibody-mediated gene transfer into bone-marrow immature hematopoietic cells

Efficient gene transfer into immature hematopoietic cells, which is considered to be a basic requirement in somatic gene therapy for genetic diseases, may also be of clinical usefulness for gene therapy of a broad range of conditions associated with acquired diseases such as cancer and infectious disorders (reviewed in Heim, 2000). The ability to deliver and to induce the expression of exogenous genes may indeed enable the performance of adequate biological manipulations of the hematopoietic stem/progenitor compartment. For example, *in vivo* targeted transfection of specific subsets of immature hematopoietic cells might help to sustain hematopoietic recovery from bone marrow aplasia by providing local production of growth factors.

Table 7.2. Number of CD34+ colonies 7 days following transfection.

Culture medium	conjugate	
	Control conjugate	anti-CD117-pIL3 conjugate
+ IL-3	97.6 ±11.7*	97 ±22
- IL-3	24 ±10.24	72.3 ±10.7

10^3 transfected CD34+ cells were cultured in methylcellulose in the presence or in the absence of IL-3. Colony (aggregates of more than 40 cells) numbers were evaluated under inverted light microscope. The data are representative of two independent experiments and are the mean of triplicate determinations ± S.D. * indicates statistically significant differences by Student's t-test analysis; $p<0.05$ as compared to cells treated with control conjugate (G250-pIL3) cultured without IL-3.

In this view, we tackled specific hematopoietic cell targeting using anti-CD117 (c-kit) Abs covalently coupled to IL-3-encoding plasmid vector {Chapel, 1999}. CD117 mAb was a good choice given its expression on a CD34+ human hematopoietic subpopulation and its ability to internalized upon binding to its ligand (Wagemaker, 1995). Targeted-gene transfer through CD117 was assayed in CD117+/CD34+ cell subset. *In vitro* cell marking with enhanced green fluorescent protein (*EGFP*) gene was first used to assess the efficiency of the transfer. Experiments were performed using CD34+ cells treated with anti-CD117-p*EGFP* conjugate and plated in methylcellulose with exogenous growth factor. After a 3-week culture, microcytometric analysis of these cells revealed 10% EGFP+ colonies (**Figure 7.5**). Then, since IL-3 has been shown to support the growth of the immature hematopoietic subpopulation (Sato, 1993), we decided to deliver human *IL-3* gene in order to evaluate the feasibility of the technique in transferring gene of functional significance and to study the biological effect of IL-3 produced upon gene transfer on the targeted population. We demonstrated that our approach allowed a transient IL-3 production in targeted cells (Chapel, 1999), leading to cell proliferation and more valuable, to the generation of CD34+ colonies even in the absence of exogenous growth factor (**Table 7.2**).

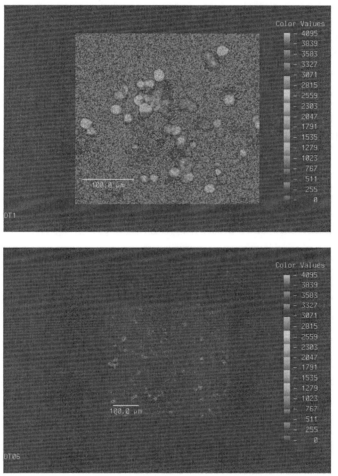

Figure 7.5 EGFP transfer into CD34+ human cells through CD117 surface Ag. (**upper picture**) cells transfected with anti-CD117=EGFP vector, (**lower picture**) transfected with EGFP gene alone.

Finally, we validated these *in vitro* results in an *in vivo* model, whereby mouse CD117+ bone-marrow cells were targeted with a vector carrying the human IL-3 encoding gene intravenously injected. As shown in **Figure 7.6**, 8 days following the last injection of the conjugates, PCR analyses of human IL-3 were positive only in bone-marrow cells from mice receiving the entire vector Taking into account all controls, PCR analysis of tissues also evidenced the specific targeting of the hematopoietic system since brain, liver and lungs were negative. Only the spleen of mice receiving IL-3 cDNA conjugated to anti-CD117 mAb and kidneys of control animals receiving either unconjugated IL-3 cDNA and anti-CD117 mAb or IL-3 cDNA conjugated to an irrelevant anti-G250 mAb, were positive in PCR. A rapid elimination of plasmid present in whole blood was observed, suggesting that these tissues were not contaminated by blood circulating plasmid. In parallel, we were able to detect circulating human IL-3 in serum of mice receiving the entire vector, only (Chapel, in preparation). However, bone-marrow cells removed from these transfected mice did not survive in long-term culture without addition of exogenous growth factor, suggesting the lost of the transgene.

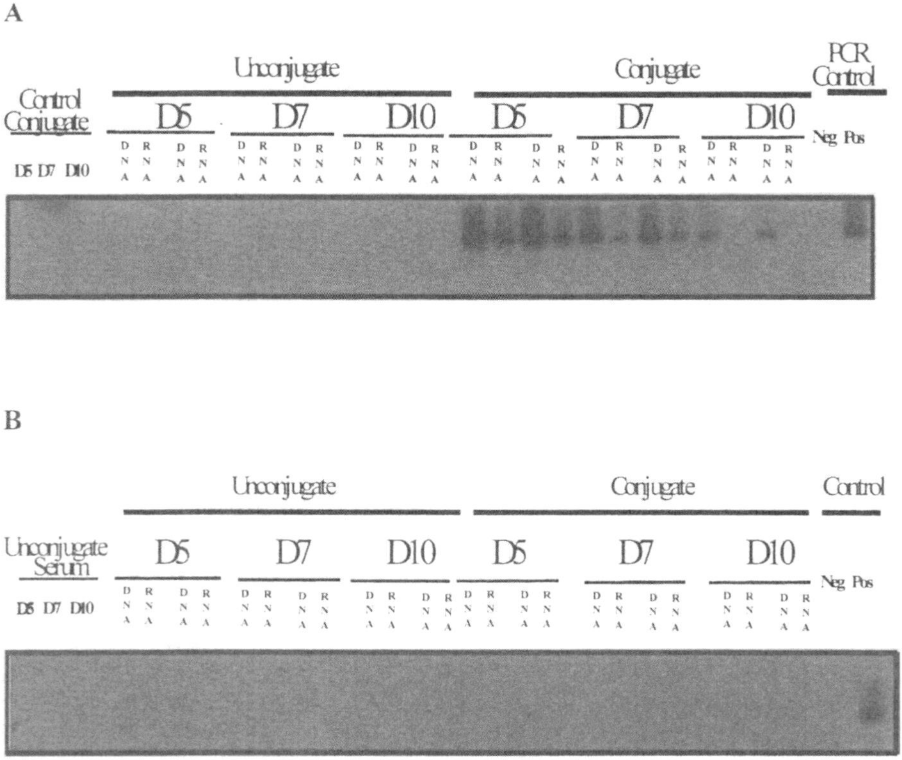

A

B

Figure 7.6 Nested PCR detection of pIL3 plasmid (A) in bone marrow and (B) in mononuclear peripheral blood cells different days after injection of theCD117mAb conjugated to human IL-3 (conjugate) or anti-CD117 Abs and human IL-3 (unconjugate).

3. CONCLUSIONS

In clinical and outpatient routine, gene therapy nowadays are still limited to rather few approaches. However, medical routine will soon be enriched by the availability of more sophisticated tools allowing specific gene delivery. As such, the availability of many mAbs directed to a wide varieties of targets will definitively enlarged the choice of disease to be treated by targeted gene therapy. Our mAb-mediated gene delivery system may prove useful and safe for numerous clinical applications of gene transfer in oncology, whereby a stable genetic modification is not required, in contrast to the gene therapy approaches for genetic diseases. Several parameters contribute to the efficiency and specificity of our system such as the internalisation of the antigen targeted, the choice of the transgene used, the tissues targeted, the conformation of the conjugate. As a caveat, it should be noted that both increasing regulatory rules, costs and practical obstacles will probably limit the use of these novel approaches to severe diseases of the economically privileged classed in Western countries. Therefore, there is a need for the search for more simple molecules using genetic engineering comprising DNA sequences and Ab-derived fragments. Finally, as we tried to illustrate in this chapter, the Cassandra who too quickly announced the death of mAbs should have in mind that *Science consists in going from an astonishment to another one* (Aristote ~ 388 AJC).

REFERENCES

Angevin, E., L. Glukhova, C. Pavon, A. Chassevent, M. J. Terrier-Lacombe, A. F. Goguel, J. Bougaran, P. Ardouin, B. H. Court, J. L. Perrin, G. Vallancien, F. Triebel, and B. Escudier. 1999. Human renal cell carcinoma xenografts in SCID mice: tumorigenicity correlates with a poor clinical prognosis. *Lab Invest 79:879.*

Arafat, W. O., et al. 2000. An adenovirus encoding proapoptotic Bax induces apoptosis and enhances the radiation effect in human ovarian cancer. *Mol Ther 1:545.*

Bartlett, J. S., J. Kleinschmidt, R. C. Boucher, and R. J. Samulski. 1999. Targeted adeno-associated virus vector transduction of nonpermissive cells mediated by a bispecific F(ab'gamma)2 antibody. *Nat Biotechnol 17:181.*

Chapel, A., P. Poncet, T. M. A. Neildez-Nguyen, J. Vétillard, N. Brouard, C. Goupy, G. Chavanel, F. Hirsch, and D. Thierry. 1999. Targeted transfection of IL-3 gene into primary human hematopoietic progenitor cells through the c-kit receptor. *Exp Hematol 27:250.*

Déas, O., E. Angevin, C. Cherbonnier, A. Senik, B. Charpentier, J. P. Levillain, E. Oosterwijk, F. Hirsch, and A. Durrbach. 2002. In vivo-targeted gene delivery using antibody-based nonviral vector. *Hum Gene Ther 13:1101.*

Dürrbach, A., E. Angevin, P. Poncet, M. Rouleau, G. Chavanel, A. Chapel, D. Thierry, A. Gorter, R. Hirsch, B. Charpentier, A. Senik, and F. Hirsch. 1999. The antibody-mediated endocytosis of G250 tumor-associated antigen allows targeted gene transfer to human renal-cell carcinoma in vitro. *Cancer Gene Ther 6:564.*

Erbacher, P., T. Bettinger, P. Belguise-Valladier, S. Zou. J. L. Coll. J. P. Behr, and J. S. Remy. 1999. Transfection and physical properties of various saccharide. poly(ethylene glycol), and antibody-derivatized polyethylenimines (PEI). *J Gene Med 1:210.*

Goud, B., P. Legrain, and G. Buttin. 1988. Antibody-mediated binding of a murine ecotropic moloney retroviral vector to human cells allows internalization but not the establishment of the proviral state. *Virology 163:251.*

Heim, D. A., and C. E. Dunbar. 2000. Hematopoietic stem cell gene therapy: towards clinically significant gene transfer efficiency. *Immunol Rev 178:29.*

Henkart, P. A. 1996. ICE family proteases: mediators of all apoptotic cell death? *Immunity 4:195.*

Hirsch, F., P. Poncet, S. Freeman, R. E. Gress, D. H. Sachs, P. Druet, and R. Hirsch. 1993. Antifection: a new method for targeted gene transfection. *Transpl Proc 25:138.*

Kohler, G., and C. Milstein. 1975. Continuous cultures of fused cells secreting antibody of predefined specificity. *Nature 256:495.*

Knudson, C. M., and S. J. Korsmeyer. 1997. *Bcl-2* and *Bax* function independently to regulate cell death. *Nature Genetics 16:358.*

Mastrobattista, E., R. H. Kapel, M. H. Eggenhuisen, P. J. Roholl, D. J. Crommelin, W. E. Hennink, and G. Storm. 2001. Lipid-coated polyplexes for targeted gene delivery to ovarian carcinoma cells. *Cancer Gene Ther 8:405.*

Maurice, M., E. Verhoeyen, P. Salmon, D. Trono, S. J. Russell, and F. L. Cosset. 2002. Efficient gene transfer into human primary blood lymphocytes by surface-engineered lentiviral vectors that display a T cell-activating polypeptide. *Blood 99:2342.*

Mulders, P., R. Figlin, J. B. deKernion, R. Wiltrout, M. Linehan, D. Parkinson, W. deWolf, and A. Belldegrun. 1997. Renal cell carcinoma: recent progress and future directions. *Cancer Res 57:5189.*

O'Neill, M. M., C. A. Kennedy, R. W. Barton, and R. J. Tatake. 2001. Receptor-mediated gene delivery to human peripheral blood mononuclear cells using anti-CD3 antibody coupled to polyethylenimine. *Gene Ther 8:362.*

Oosterwijk, E., D. J. Ruitter, P. J. Hoedemaeker, E. K. J. Pauwels, U. Jonas, J. Zwartendijck, and S. O. Warnaar. 1986. Monoclonal antibody G250 recognizes a determinant present in renal-cell carcinoma and absent from normal kidney. *Int J Cancer 38:489.*

Oosterwijk, E., F. M. J. Debruyne, and J. A. Schalken. 1995. The use of monoclonal antibody G250 in the therapy of renal-cell carcinoma. *Semin Oncol 22:34.*

Pelegrin, M., M. Marin, D. Noel, and M. Piechaczyk. 1998. Genetically engineered antibodies in gene transfer and gene therapy. *Hum Gene Ther 9:2165.*

Perales, J. C., T. Ferkol, H. Beegen, O. D. Ratnoff, and R. W. Hanson. 1994. Gene transfer *in vivo*: Sustained expression and regulation of genes introduced into the liver by receptor-targeted uptake. *Proc Natl Acad Sci USA 91:4086.*

Poncet, P., A. Panczak, C. Goupy, K. Gustafsson, C. Blanpied, G. Chavanel, R. Hirsch, and F. Hirsch. 1996. Antifection: an antibody-mediated method to introduce genes into lymphoid cells in vitro and in vivo. *Gene Ther 3:731.*

Roselli, M., F. Guadagni, O. Buonomo, A. Belardi, P. Ferroni, A. Diodati, D. Anselmi, C. Cipriani, C. U. Casciani, J. Greiner, and J. Schlom. 1996. Tumor markers as targets for selective diagnostic and therapeutic procedures. *Anticancer Res 16:2187.*

Sato, N., C. Caux, T. Kitamura, Y. Watanabe, K. Arai, J. Banchereau, and A. Miyajima. 1993. Expression and factor-dependent modulation of the interleukin-3 receptor subunits on human hematopoietic cells. *Blood 82:752.*

Schwarzenberger, P., S. E. Spence, J. M. Gooya, D. Michiel, D. T. Curiel, F. W. Ruscetti, and J. R. Keller. 1996. Targeted gene transfer to human hematopoietic progenitor cell lines through the c-kit receptor. *Blood 67:472.*

Shi, N., and W. M. Pardridge. 2000. Noninvasive gene targeting to the brain. *Proc Natl Acad Sci U S A 97:7567.*

Tai, Y. T., T. Strobel, D. Kufe, and S. A. Cannistra. 1999. In vivo cytotoxicity of ovarian cancer cells through tumor-selective expression of the BAX gene. *Cancer Res 59:2121.*

Templeton, N. S., D. D. Lasic, P. M. Frederik, H. H. Strey, D. D. Roberts, and G. N. Pavlakis. 1997. Improved DNA: liposome complexes for increased systemic delivery and gene expression. *Nat Biotechnol 15:647.*

Tsuruta, Y., M. Mandai, I. Konishi, H. Kuroda, T. Kusakari, Y. Yura, A. A. Hamid, I. Tamura, M. Kariya, and S. Fujii. 2001. Combination effect of adenovirus-mediated pro-apoptotic bax gene transfer with cisplatin or paclitaxel treatment in ovarian cancer cell lines. *Eur J Cancer 37:531.*

Wagemaker, G., K. J. Neelis, and A. W. Wognum. 1995. Surface markers and growth factor receptors of immature hemopoietic stem cell subsets. *Stem Cells 13 Suppl 1:165.*

Wagner, E., M. Zenke, M. Cotten, H. Beug, and M. L. Birnstiel. 1990. Transferrin-polycation conjugates as carriers for DNA uptake into cells. *Proc Natl Acad Sci USA 87:3410.*

Wang, R. F., and S. A. Rosenberg. 1999. Human tumor antigens for cancer vaccine development. *Immunol Rev 170:85.*

Weichselbaum, R. R., and D. Kufe. 1997. Gene therapy of cancer. *Lancet 349:10.*

Wickham, T. J. 2000. Targeting adenovirus. *Gene Ther 7:110.*

Xu, L., C. C. Huang, W. Huang, W. H. Tang, A. Rait, Y. Z. Yin, I. Cruz, L. M. Xiang, K. F. Pirollo, and E. H. Chang. 2002. Systemic tumor-targeted gene delivery by anti-transferrin receptor scFv-immunoliposomes. *Mol Cancer Ther 1:337.*

Zenke, M., P. Steinlein, E. Wagner, M. Cotten, H. Beug, and M. L. Birnstiel. 1990. Receptor-mediated endocytosis of transferrin-polycation conjugates: an efficient way to introduce DNA into hematopoietic cells. *Proc Natl Acad Sci USA 87:3655.*

Zhang, Y., H. Jeong Lee, R. J. Boado, and W. M. Pardridge. 2002. Receptor-mediated delivery of an antisense gene to human brain cancer cells. *J Gene Med 4:183.*

Chapter 8

INTRABODIES: DEVELOPMENT AND APPLICATION IN FUNCTIONAL GENOMICS AND THERAPY

Alcide Barberis, Adrian Auf Der Maur, Kathrin Tissot, and Peter Lichtlen
ESBATech AG, Wagistr. 21, 8952 Zürich-Schlieren, Switzerland (www.esbatech.com)

1.   INTRODUCTION

The human genome project has led to the identification of a large number of genes and respective proteins, thus providing the pharmaceutical industry with thousands of new potential drug targets, most of which function in intracellular compartments (Lander *et al.*, 2001; Venter *et al.*, 2001). This fact opens new perspectives for therapy of human diseases; however, it also demands reliable approaches for understanding the role and the function of these new genes and proteins (functional genomics) and for identifying those that can be validated as drug targets (target validation). Different experimental tools are currently used for investigating the function of these new intracellular proteins, including their potential role in disease, and for evaluating them as potential drug targets. The classical way to investigate the function of genes, and thereby determine the physiological and pathological relevance of gene products, is to interfere with their expression (Ihle, 2000). Approaches such as gene knockout, antisense oligonucleotide or RNA interference (RNAi) are currently used to study gene and protein function and to validate candidate drug targets by analysing the effects of their deletion. One limitation of all these techniques is that they eliminate all functions of a target gene product at once, thus making it difficult to dissect potentially distinct roles of different domains and to mimic the effects of a small molecule that presumably will act at a specific domain of the protein

(Kamb and Caponigro, 2001). Intrabodies, *i.e.* antibody fragments expressed within the cell, present an attractive alternative for directly modulating protein function *in vivo.* In particular, intrabodies can be used to target specific domains of a protein and perform so-called "protein-domain knockouts", thus allowing the dissection of the varied functions of multi-domain proteins (Lichtlen *et al.*, 2002).

The idea of validating drug targets at the protein level harbours conceptual advantages. Firstly, by aiming at the protein one acts on the potential target directly. Moreover, by specifically blocking the function of protein domains, the action of highly specific drugs can be mimicked and their biological effects anticipated. It has become evident that highly specific drugs are associated with fewer side effects than non-specific drugs, thus underlying the importance of studying the function of specific domains of protein targets (Ihle, 2000). A remarkable example for this concept has been provided by Rao and collaborators (Aramburu *et al.*, 1999). In this study it was shown that a peptide capable of selectively blocking the NFAT-binding site of calcineurin, the molecular target of the immunosuppressive drugs cyclosporine A and FK506, efficiently inhibited the expression of NFAT-dependent cytokines in T cells. At the same time, other cytokines, whose expression is dependent on non-NFAT-mediated calcineurin activity, were not affected by the inhibitory peptide. Cyclosporine A and FK506 inhibit the activation of all genes that are dependent on calcineurin activity and do not discriminate between those that require the action of NFAT from those that do not. Their action leads to effective immunosuppression but also to severe side effects, such as progressive loss of renal function, neurotoxicity or increased risk of malignancy (Ruhlmann and Nordheim, 1997). As these side effects are assigned to the inhibition of non-NFAT-mediated actions of calcineurin, Rao and colleagues have given a nice example on how targeting protein domains can be useful for development of therapeutic agents that are potentially less toxic than current drugs because of their higher level of specificity. The advantage of dealing with a protein target directly and the potential to functionally neutralize specific protein domains taken together with the high degree of specificity and affinity that antibodies can show have made the use of intrabodies for intracellular applications more and more important in the fields of functional genomics and target validation (Cattaneo and Biocca, 1997).

2.   DEVELOPMENT OF INTRABODIES

Intrabodies have been generally derived from specific monoclonal antibodies or from antibody fragments (most commonly the single-chain Fv (scFv) format) that were initially selected for specific antigen-binding activity by *in vitro* techniques (phage- or ribosome-display) and subsequently tested for their performance as modulators of antigen function within eukaryotic cells (Pörtner-Taliana *et al.*, 2000; Visintin *et al.*, 1999; Wörn *et al.*, 2000). This procedure does not ensure that the *in vitro*-isolated antibodies also bind their cognate antigen in the cytoplasm of a cell. In fact, the cytoplasm is a non-physiological environment for antibodies, which naturally work outside cells. The reducing conditions within the cytoplasm prevent the formation of the highly conserved disulfide bonds, which guarantee proper folding and stability of antibody frameworks also in the scFv format. Thus, the intracellular expression of antibodies is generally confronted with difficulties concerning folding, stability and solubility (tendency to aggregate) (Wörn *et al.*, 2000). For this reason most antibodies and antibody fragments have been found to be inactive inside eukaryotic cells (Biocca *et al.*, 1995; Martineau *et al.*, 1998). As a consequence of these facts, highly stable and soluble antibody frameworks, which can fold even in the absence of the disulfide bonds and do not undergo aggregation, are required for the application of intrabodies as potential modulators of protein function *in vivo* (Mössner *et al.*, 2001; Wörn and Plückthun, 2001).

Since only a small fraction of a typical scFv antibody library will generally have sufficient stability for intracellular applications (Pörtner-Taliana *et al.*, 2000), one approach to obtain a much higher number of functional intrabodies can be provided by constructing randomized hypervariable loop libraries on antibody frameworks that have been pre-selected for high stability and solubility in an intracellular environment (Auf der Maur *et al.*, 2002). The few antibodies that have been found to function in an intracellular environment and that have been characterized for their biophysical properties have generally shown a high degree of stability and solubility (Auf der Maur *et al.*, 2002; Wörn and Plückthun, 2001). The sequence requirements that make antibody frameworks very stable such that they might also function in an intracellular environment are only now emerging (Ewert *et al.*, 2003). At ESBATech, we have developed a simple technology, called "Quality Control", which allows rapid selection of stable and soluble antibody frameworks *in vivo* without the requirement or knowledge of antigens, (Auf der Maur *et al.*, 2001).

The "Quality Control" system to identify intracellular stable and soluble antibody frameworks (most commonly scFvs) is based on the hypothesis that stability and solubility (and therefore the activity) of a fusion protein composed of a constant, selectable marker fused to, for example, an scFv is determined by the quality of the scFv moiety. To test this hypothesis, and to prove the principle of the method, a number of well-characterized scFvs were fused to a marker protein, which, when expressed in an active form, can specifically activate expression of selectable reporter genes in yeast (Auf der Maur *et al.*, 2001). Figure 8.1 depicts the principle of our method as tested with the marker protein composed of a peptide (P) linked to a transcriptional activation domain (AD).

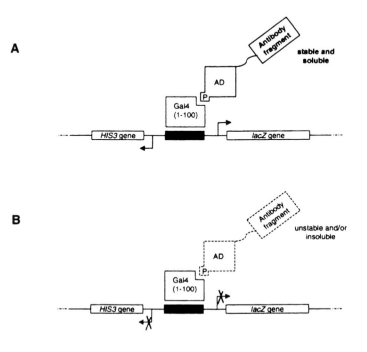

Figure 8.1. The "Quality Control" system for the antigen-independent selection of intracellular stable antibody frameworks. Antibody fragments are fused to a selectable marker protein comprising a transcriptional activation domain (AD) and a peptide derived from Gal11P (P), which can mediate the specific interaction with the DNA-bound Gal4 (1-100) fragment. The basic concept of the "Quality Control" system is that the activity of the entire fusion protein carrying the selectable marker is dependent on the stability and solubility of the antibody moiety. A: A fusion protein carrying a stable and soluble antibody fragment is tethered to DNA via the Gal4(1-100)-Gal11P interaction where it activates transcription of the divergently oriented *lacZ* and *HIS3* reporter genes (bent arrows). B: Unstable and/or insoluble antibody moieties lead to inactivation of the entire fusion protein (dashed lines), thus impeding activation of transcription of the reporter genes (crossed arrows).

The peptide (P) was derived from the mutant form of the yeast protein Gal11 called Gal11P. It has been previously shown that only the mutant Gal11P peptide, but not the wild-type sequence, specifically interacts with the dimerization region of the DNA-binding Gal4 fragment comprising the first 100 amino acids (Barberis and Gaudreau, 1998; Barberis *et al.*, 1995). The activation domain (AD) of Gal4 is known to activate transcription when tethered to DNA via protein-protein interactions (Fields and Sternglanz,

1994). According to the hypothesis outlined above, a fusion protein bearing a soluble and stable antibody fragment should be tethered to DNA via the Gal4(1-100)-Gal11P interaction and, thus, activate transcription of the reporter genes, whereas an unstable and/or insoluble antibody fragment should render the entire fusion protein inactive (Fig. 1). The divergently oriented *lacZ* and *HIS3* reporter genes allow quantification of the level of gene activation and positive growth selection on selective media, respectively (Auf der Maur *et al.*, 2001). The possibility to select for antigen-independent cell growth stimulation is particularly useful for screening naïve antibody libraries fused to the marker protein in order to select frameworks that are stable and soluble in an intracellular environment. This technology also allows improving the intracellular performance of an existing binder, which might be poorly stable or prone to aggregation, through a "framework evolution process" by random diversification of the primary sequence and subsequent growth selection in yeast. It is worth noting that the assessment of solubility and stability of a recombinant antibody fragment by means of cellular expression is not necessarily restricted to transcriptional activity. These properties can also be tested with alternative types of "constant markers", which provide certain selectable activity that is dependent on the stability and solubility of the intrabody.

In our laboratories, analysis of more than 50 framework sequences that were selected in the "Quality Control" system showed that they belong to subfamilies of variable domains with a track record of high stability and good folding properties *in vitro* (Ewert *et al.*, 2003). In agreement with this sequence analysis, the biophysical characterization of some of the selected frameworks *in vitro* confirmed their high degree of stability and solubility under various conditions. Moreover, production of these antibody fragments from bacteria gave significantly higher yields than those obtained with average antibodies, *i.e.* over 100 mg proteins per liter culture.

Frameworks selected in the "Quality Control" system subsequently serve as scaffolds or acceptor backbones to construct "complementarity determining region" (CDR) libraries by randomization of one or more hypervariable loops. Such antibody libraries based on "super-stable frameworks" are then screened to identify antigen-specific binders either in a phage display format or again in yeast in a modified two-hybrid system (Fields and Sternglanz, 1994), in which purification of the antigen is not required (Auf der Maur *et al.*, 2002). In this assay, the antibody fragment is linked to a transcriptional activation domain, while the target antigen is linked to a DNA-binding domain. A specific interaction between the antibody fusion protein and the antigen leads to expression of reporter genes, thus allowing an efficient screen of intrabody libraries by yeast cell growth selection (Auf der Maur *et al.*, 2002; Pörtner-Taliana *et al.*, 2000; Visintin *et al.*, 2002; Visintin *et al.*, 1999).

The "Quality Control" system to select intrabody frameworks, taken together with the antigen-specific screening of libraries constructed on such "super-stable frameworks", open new possibilities to obtain highly performing intrabodies suitable for intracellular applications. However, one problem for the efficient screening of large libraries in yeast is caused by the comparatively low transformation efficiency that can be achieved in this organism. In contrast, *in vitro* screening techniques such as ribosome display (Hanes and Plückthun, 1997) or mRNA display (Wilson *et al.*, 2001) can explore libraries that reach a complexity of approximately 10^{13} to 10^{14}. Thus, the low transformation efficiency of yeast appears to be disadvantageous for screening highly complex CDR libraries. In order to solve this problem, we apply the following strategy. Given that a typical intrabody library is based on a framework that is optimised for the reducing environment of the cytoplasm and that the antigen-antibody interaction is selected *in vivo*, it is conceivable that at least weak binders can be identified from less complex libraries. Thus, we first randomise just a few but crucial amino acids, starting for example with the CDR3 of the variable heavy chain, which is the most important antigen-binding sequence. Thereby, the library presents a complexity that can still be completely screened in yeast. Since the chance to immediately isolate a high-affinity binder is rather low, it is reasonable to follow a stepwise approach (Auf der Maur *et al.*, 2002). Thus, in a first screening round low affinity binders are isolated while in a second round randomisation of another CDR is performed and the derived library is again selected *in vivo* under increased selection stringency.

3.   APPLICATIONS OF INTRABODIES

3.1   In functional genomics

Intrabodies have been shown to interfere with protein function in a number of ways, affording them great potential for the use in functional genomics and target validation. Intrabodies directed against specific domains can for example block protein-protein interactions. In collaboration with the laboratory of Dr. Andreas Plückthun, we have shown that intracellular stable single-chain antibodies targeted against the dimerization domain of the yeast transcriptional activator Gcn4 significantly reduced its activation function (Wörn *et al.*, 2000). Gcn4 belongs to the family of proteins with a leucine zipper dimerization domain that is required for efficient and sequence specific DNA binding (Hope and Struhl, 1987). Two point mutations in the leucine zipper motif that prevented dimer formation *in vitro* (Leder *et al.*, 1995) also abolished the transcription activation function of Gcn4 *in vivo* (Wörn *et al.*, 2000). Our results show that intracellular single-chain antibodies directed against the Gcn4 leucine zipper, which have been shown to interfere with dimerization of this protein *in vitro* (Berger *et al.*, 1999), could reduce activation of a Gcn4-dependent gene to various extents down to about 15% (Wörn *et al.*, 2000). The different inhibitory effects of these various intrabodies directed against the Gcn4 dimerization domain correlated with their stability and solubility (Wörn *et al.*, 2000), thus indicating the importance of these parameters for designing or selecting effective intrabodies.

Domain-specific intrabodies have also been shown to interfere with protein-DNA interactions. An intracellular scFv derived from a monoclonal antibody, which was characterized for its ability to specifically prevent DNA binding by the human transcription factor ATF-1 *in vitro*, inhibited ATF-1-activated transcription *in vivo* as well as ATF-1 dependent tumorigenicity and metastatic potential of transfected melanoma cells in mice (Jean *et al.*, 2000).

In addition to blocking protein activities, and in contrast to gene or RNA knockout techniques, intrabodies directed against specific domains can also have agonistic effects, thus stimulating or even restoring target protein function. For example, two intrabodies able to associate with p53 and to restore DNA binding activity of some p53 mutants *in vitro* were shown to recover the transcriptional activity of these p53 mutants in transfected tumor cells (Caron de Fromentel *et al.*, 1999).

A number of studies have demonstrated the ability of intrabodies to interfere with cellular processes by relocating specific proteins so as to take them away from their natural site of action. For example, redirecting the cytoplasmic Tau protein to the nucleus neutralized its function (Visintin *et al.*, 2002). Diverting Ras from its natural location by Ras-specific intrabodies also caused neutralization of its function (Lener *et al.*, 2000). It is worth noting that this particular antibody was shown to have no effect on Ras in an *in vitro* system and, therefore, its neutralizing effect *in vivo* was solely due to its ability to relocate the target to a "silencing" site. A further example for this mode of action of intrabodies is provided by the results of Zhu *et al.*, who showed that relocation of Caspase 7 by nuclear-targeted specific intrabodies significantly inhibited staurosporine-induced apoptosis (Zhu *et al.*, 1999).

Intrabodies have been shown to affect intracellular protein functions in a variety of biological systems. To date, most of the data regarding the use of intrabodies to analyse protein function, as well as to test their potential therapeutic application, have been obtained from experiments performed with cultured mammalian cells (Cattaneo and Biocca, 1999; Marasco, 1997). However, the first application of intrabodies in functional genomics was established in yeast (Carlson, 1988).

In addition to their broad use in single-cell biological systems, intrabodies have also been shown to function in multicellular organisms. For example, constitutive expression in transgenic plants of an intrabody directed against a plant virus caused reduction of viral infection incidence and significantly delayed the development of symptoms (Tavladoraki *et al.*, 1993). Intrabodies have also been successfully applied in the fruit fly *Drosophila melanogaster* to functionally neutralize the transcription factor Poxn, leading to the reproduction of the poxn⁻ phenotype (Hassanzadeh *et al.*, 1998).

3.2   In therapy

Although intrabodies have not yet been used to cure human diseases, their specific biophysical properties (high stability and solubility) that allow them to function also in the adverse intracellular environment, taken together with the general characteristics of antibodies (high affinity and specificity), make them promising tools for therapeutic applications.

The most straightforward application of intrabodies in therapy studies is through intracellular expression of these proteins from genes inserted into target cells. This has been achieved by gene therapy approaches using viral vectors for gene delivery and expression. One of the most advanced applications of intrabodies in a gene therapy setting is represented by the ability of specific intrabodies to block replication of a virus in transduced human cells (Marasco, 1997; Mhashilkar *et al.*, 1995). The pioneering work of Marasco and collaborators from the Dana-Farber Cancer Institute in Boston has demonstrated the successful use of intrabodies directed against HIV-1 proteins or their functional partners in inhibiting viral replication in targeted T cells, thus making these cells permanently resistant to viral attack. In their most recent work (Bai *et al.*, 2003), these authors have shown that intrabodies binding the human hCyclin T1 protein, whose interaction with the HIV-1 Tat protein is required for efficient production of full-length viral genome, were able to inhibit Tat-mediated transactivation and HIV-1 replication in transfected human T cells. Since these intrabodies did not inhibit cellular basal transcription or cause any other apparent side effect, the results of Marasco and collaborators represent a significant step towards gene therapy strategies to treat HIV-1 infection and AIDS that are based on a so-called "intracellular immunization". Despite the success of current highly active anti-retroviral therapies (HAART) for the treatment of AIDS, a large proportion of HIV-1-infected patients become refractory to these treatments or do not tolerate for a long period of time the toxic effects of this therapy. Gene therapy through the introduction of anti-viral resistance genes into CD4+ T cells, or even more appropriately into pluripotent hematopoietic CD34+ stem cells, is one important approach that could give long term *in vivo* protection to cells that are susceptible to HIV-1.

A technique that emerged a few years ago, which has recently received increasing attention, might become an important alternative to the gene therapy approach for delivering intrabodies or other proteins inside cells. "Protein transduction", or "protein therapy", as this novel approach is called, is based on the observation that proteins fused to some particular short peptides, such as that derived from the HIV-1 Tat protein, can efficiently cross cell membranes and thus be delivered into tissues (Wadia and Dowdy, 2002). The first "protein therapy" experiments were performed with tissue culture cells in Petri dishes (Derossi *et al.*, 1996; Nagahara *et al.*, 1998). The *in vivo* breakthrough came with the work of Dowdy and collaborators, who showed that intraperitoneal injection of β-galactosidase fused to the protein transduction domain (PTD) of the HIV-1 Tat protein resulted in delivery of the biologically active hybrid protein to all tissues in mice, including the brain (Schwarze *et al.*, 1999). More recently, Ohta and collaborators have shown that a potent derivative of the antiapoptotic protein Bcl-x$_L$ fused to the Tat peptide could readily enter cultured neurons and protect them from apoptotic stimuli. More importantly, when injected intraperitoneally into gerbils, this hybrid protein efficiently prevented neuronal death triggered by transient global ischemia (Asoh *et al.*, 2002).

For the development of intrabodies as therapeutic proteins, it will be important to further study their application in gene therapy, as well as to test them as fusion proteins with transducing peptide motifs in "protein therapy" approaches. It is important to note that, while a high degree of stability and solubility of antibody fragments is absolutely required for intracellular applications in gene therapy or "protein therapy", these properties are very much desirable also for classical therapeutic applications of antibodies towards extracellular targets and as diagnostic tools (Harris, 1999; Willuda *et al.*, 1999). Moreover, high stability and solubility of these proteins greatly facilitate their expression and purification from microorganisms such as bacteria and yeast, thus lowering costs and reducing time for their production (Hudson and Souriau, 2003).

ACKNOWLEDGEMENTS

We would like to thank all the members of the Antibody Unit at ESBATech AG for fruitful discussion, and Andreas Plückthun, Arne Wörn and Christian Zahnd for their collaboration and for providing materials for the development of the "Quality Control" system.

REFERENCES

Aramburu, J., Yaffe, M. B., Lopez-Rodriguez, C., Cantley, L. C., Hogan, P. G., and Rao, A. (1999). Affinity-driven peptide selection of an NFAT inhibitor more selective than cyclosporin A. Science *285*, 2129-2133.

Asoh, S., Ohsawa, I., Mori, T., Katsura, K., Hiraide, T., Katayama, Y., Kimura, M., Ozaki, D., Yamagata, K., and Ohta, S. (2002). Protection against ischemic brain injury by protein therapeutics. Proc Natl Acad Sci U S A *99*, 17107-17112.

Auf der Maur, A., Escher, D., and Barberis, A. (2001). Antigen-independent selection of stable intracellular single-chain antibodies. FEBS Lett *508*, 407-412.

Auf der Maur, A., Zahnd, C., Fischer, F., Spinelli, S., Honegger, A., Cambillau, C., Escher, D., Pluckthun, A., and Barberis, A. (2002). Direct in vivo screening of intrabody libraries constructed on a highly stable single-chain framework. J Biol Chem *277*, 45075-45085.

Bai, J., Sui, J., Zhu, R. Y., Tallarico, A. S., Gennari, F., Zhang, D., and Marasco, W. A. (2003). Inhibition of Tat-mediated transactivation and HIV-1 replication by human anti-hCyclinT1 intrabodies. J Biol Chem *278*, 1433-1442.

Barberis, A., and Gaudreau, L. (1998). Recruitment of the RNA polymerase II holoenzyme and its implications in gene regulation. Biol Chem *379*, 1397-1405.

Barberis, A., Pearlberg, J., Simkovich, N., Farrell, S., Reinagel, P., Bamdad, C., Sigal, G., and Ptashne, M. (1995). Contact with a component of the polymerase II holoenzyme suffices for gene activation. Cell *81*, 359-368.

Berger, C., Weber-Bornhauser, S., Eggenberger, J., Hanes, J., Pluckthun, A., and Bosshard, H. R. (1999). Antigen recognition by conformational selection. FEBS Lett *450*, 149-153.

Biocca, S., Ruberti, F., Tafani, M., Pierandrei-Amaldi, P., and Cattaneo, A. (1995). Redox state of single chain Fv fragments targeted to the endoplasmic reticulum, cytosol and mitochondria. Bio/Technology *13*, 1110-1115.

Carlson, J. R. (1988). A new means of inducibly inactivating a cellular protein. Mol Cell Biol *8*, 2638-2646.

Caron de Fromentel, C., Gruel, N., Venot, C., Debussche, L., Conseiller, E., Dureuil, C., Teillaud, J. L., Tocque, B., and Bracco, L. (1999). Restoration of transcriptional activity of p53 mutants in human tumour cells by intracellular expression of anti-p53 single chain Fv fragments. Oncogene *18*, 551-557.

Cattaneo, A., and Biocca, S. (1997). Intracellular antibodies: Development and applications (New York, Springer).

Cattaneo, A., and Biocca, S. (1999). The selection of intracellular antibodies. Trends In Biotechnology *17*, 115-121.

Derossi, D., Calvet, S., Trembleau, A., Brunissen, A., Chassaing, G., and Prochiantz, A. (1996). Cell internalization of the third helix of the Antennapedia homeodomain is receptor-independent. J Biol Chem *271*, 18188-18193.

Ewert, S., Huber, T., Honegger, A., and Pluckthun, A. (2003). Biophysical properties of human antibody variable domains. J Mol Biol *325*, 531-553.

Fields, S., and Sternglanz, R. (1994). The two-hybrid system: an assay for protein-protein interactions. Trends in Genetics *10*, 286-292.

Hanes, J., and Plückthun, A. (1997). In vitro selection and evolution of functional proteins by using ribosome display. Proc Natl Acad Sci U S A *94*, 4937-4942.

Harris, B. (1999). Exploiting antibody-based technologies to manage environmental pollution. Trends Biotechnol *17*, 290-296.

Hassanzadeh, G. G., De Silva, K. S., Dambly-Chaudiere, C., Brys, L., Ghysen, A., Hamers, R., Muyldermans, S., and De Baetselier, P. (1998). Isolation and characterization of single-chain Fv genes encoding antibodies specific for Drosophila Poxn protein. FEBS Lett *437*, 75-80.

Hope, I. A., and Struhl, K. (1987). GCN4, a eukaryotic transcriptional activator protein, binds as a dimer to target DNA. Embo J *6*, 2781-2784.

Hudson, P. J., and Souriau, C. (2003). Engineered antibodies. Nat Med *9*, 129-134.

Ihle, J. N. (2000). The challenges of translating knockout phenotypes into gene function. Cell *102*, 131-134.

Jean, D., Tellez, C., Huang, S., Davis, D. W., Bruns, C. J., McConkey, D. J., Hinrichs, S. H., and Bar-Eli, M. (2000). Inhibition of tumor growth and metastasis of human melanoma by intracellular anti-ATF-1 single chain Fv fragment. Oncogene *19*, 2721-2730.

Kamb, A., and Caponigro, G. (2001). Peptide inhibitors expressed in vivo. Curr Opin Chem Biol *5*, 74-77.

Lander, E. S., Linton, L. M., Birren, B., Nusbaum, C., Zody, M. C., Baldwin, J., Devon, K., Dewar, K., Doyle, M., FitzHugh, W., *et al.* (2001). Initial sequencing and analysis of the human genome. Nature *409*, 860-921.

Leder, L., Berger, C., Bornhauser, S., Wendt, H., Ackermann, F., Jelesarov, I., and Bosshard, H. R. (1995). Spectroscopic, calorimetric, and kinetic demonstration of conformational adaptation in peptide-antibody recognition. Biochemistry *34*, 16509-16518.

Lener, M., Horn, I. R., Cardinale, A., Messina, S., Nielsen, U. B., Rybak, S. M., Hoogenboom, H. R., Cattaneo, A., and Biocca, S. (2000). Diverting a protein from its cellular location by intracellular antibodies. The case of p21Ras. Eur J Biochem *267*, 1196-1205.

Lichtlen, P., Auf der Maur, A., and Barberis, A. (2002). Target validation through protein-domain knockout: applications of intracellularly stable single-chain antibodies. TARGETS *1*, 37-44.

Marasco, W. A. (1997). Intrabodies: turning the humoral immune system outside in for intracellular immunization. Gene Ther *4*, 11-15.

Martineau, P., Jones, P., and Winter, G. (1998). Expression of an antibody fragment at high levels in the bacterial cytoplasm. J Mol Biol *280*, 117-127.

Mhashilkar, A. M., Bagley, J., Chen, S. Y., Szilvay, A. M., Helland, D. G., and Marasco, W. A. (1995). Inhibition of HIV-1 Tat-mediated LTR transactivation and HIV-1 infection by anti-Tat single chain intrabodies. EMBO Journal *14*, 1542-1551.

Mössner, E., Koch, H., and Plückthun, A. (2001). Fast selection of antibodies without antigen purification: adaptation of the protein fragment complementation assay to select antigen-antibody pairs. J Mol Biol *308*, 115-122.

Nagahara, H., Vocero-Akbani, A. M., Snyder, E. L., Ho, A., Latham, D. G., Lissy, N. A., Becker-Hapak, M., Ezhevsky, S. A., and Dowdy, S. F. (1998). Transduction of full-length TAT fusion proteins into mammalian cells: TAT-p27Kip1 induces cell migration. Nat Med *4*, 1449-1452.

Pörtner-Taliana, A., Russell, M., Froning, K. J., Budworth, P. R., Comiskey, J. D., and Hoeffler, J. P. (2000). In vivo selection of single-chain antibodies using a yeast two-hybrid system. J Immunol Methods *238*, 161-172.

Ruhlmann, A., and Nordheim, A. (1997). Effects of the immunosuppressive drugs CsA and FK506 on intracellular signalling and gene regulation. Immunobiology *198*, 192-206.

Schwarze, S. R., Ho, A., Vocero-Akbani, A., and Dowdy, S. F. (1999). In vivo protein transduction: delivery of a biologically active protein into the mouse. Science *285*, 1569-1572.

Tavladoraki, P., Benvenuto, E., Trinca, S., De Martinis, D., Cattaneo, A., and Galeffi, P. (1993). Transgenic plants expressing a functional single-chain Fv antibody are specifically protected from virus attack. Nature *366*, 469-472.

Venter, J. C., Adams, M. D., Myers, E. W., Li, P. W., Mural, R. J., Sutton, G. G., Smith, H. O., Yandell, M., Evans, C. A., Holt, R. A., *et al.* (2001). The sequence of the human genome. Science *291*, 1304-1351.

Visintin, M., Settanni, G., Maritan, A., Graziosi, S., Marks, J. D., and Cattaneo, A. (2002). The Intracellular Antibody Capture Technology (IACT): Towards a Consensus Sequence for Intracellular Antibodies. J Mol Biol *317*, 73-83.

Visintin, M., Tse, E., Axelson, H., Rabbitts, T. H., and Cattaneo, A. (1999). Selection of antibodies for intracellular function using a two-hybrid in vivo system. Proc Natl Acad Sci U S A *96*, 11723-11728.

Wadia, J. S., and Dowdy, S. F. (2002). Protein transduction technology. Curr Opin Biotechnol *13*, 52-56.

Willuda, J., Honegger, A., Waibel, R., Schubiger, P. A., Stahel, R., Zangemeister-Wittke, U., and Plückthun, A. (1999). High thermal stability is essential for tumor targeting of antibody fragments: engineering of a humanized anti-epithelial glycoprotein-2 (epithelial cell adhesion molecule) single-chain Fv fragment. Cancer Res *59*, 5758-5767.

Wilson, D. S., Keefe, A. D., and Szostak, J. W. (2001). The use of mRNA display to select high-affinity protein-binding peptides. Proc Natl Acad Sci U S A *98*, 3750-3755.

Wörn, A., Auf der Maur, A., Escher, D., Honegger, A., Barberis, A., and Plückthun, A. (2000). Correlation between in vitro stability and in vivo performance of anti-GCN4 intrabodies as cytoplasmic inhibitors. J Biol Chem *275*, 2795-2803.

Wörn, A., and Plückthun, A. (2001). Stability engineering of antibody single-chain Fv fragments. J Mol Biol *305*, 989-1010.

Zhu, Q., Zeng, C., Huhalov, A., Yao, J., Turi, T. G., Danley, D., Hynes, T., Cong, Y., DiMattia, D., Kennedy, S., *et al.* (1999). Extended half-life and elevated steady-state level of a single-chain Fv intrabody are critical for specific intracellular retargeting of its antigen, caspase-7. J Immunol Methods *231*, 207-222.

Chapter 9

EXPRESSION OF RECOMBINANT ANTIBODIES BY TUMOUR CELLS: ON ROAD TO ANTI-TUMOUR THERAPY

Emmanuelle Bonnin[*], and Jean-Luc Teillaud[*]
[*]Unité INSERM 255, Centre de Recherches Biomédicales des Cordeliers, 15 rue de l'Ecole de Médecine, 75270 Paris cedex 06, France

1. INTRODUCTION

Monoclonal antibodies are attractive tools for cancer therapy and have now come of age as therapeutics. Their exquisite specificity, combined with their ability to activate potent effector functions makes them an ideal tool for cancer therapy. Depending on their classes and subclasses, antibodies can activate complement and/or trigger effector functions such as Antibody-Dependent Cell Cytotoxicity (ADCC) following interactions with the receptors for the Fc region of IgG or IgA (FcγR and FcαR). Over the last decade, therapeutic antibodies have moved to the forefront of protein drug development, mostly due to the formidable capacity to engineer their immunogenicity, their affinity and their functions (Mehren et al., 2003). Therapeutic monoclonal antibodies are currently being used to target either soluble circulating molecules such as cytokines or cell surface antigens following systemic delivery. They also represent exciting tools for the targeted delivery of drugs, enzymes, and toxins at the site of the tumours. In addition, antibody-based radio-immunotherapy (RIT) should make it possible to circumvent the limitation of the treatment of solid tumours with antibodies due to the weak penetration of intact antibody molecules.

The specific targeting of intracellular molecules involved in a variety of cellular functions altered in tumour cells has been a major goal of the pharmaceutical industry for several decades. However, it is clear that the search for new chemical compounds that exhibit an exquisite specificity and a high affinity for intracellular targets has become an extremely difficult task, a quest for the Holy Graal. Huge libraries of chemical compounds have been screened using High-Throughput Screening (HTS), but the number of drugs that have been then developed and marketed are limited if one consider the efforts made.

By contrast, molecules that were rationally designed, based on structural and functional studies of mutated proteins in tumour cells, such as STI-571, are very promising on a clinical point of view. Thus, the idea that antibodies, that are naturally "rationally designed" by the immune system to bind target antigens with high specificity and affinity, could be also used as intracellular drugs has emerged in the early 90's (Biocca *et al.*, 1990; Marasco *et al.*, 1993).

The intracellular expression of recombinant antibodies has enormous potential advantages (Cochet *et al.*, 1998a; Marasco, 2001; Cohen, 2002). First, they can be expressed under short fragments such as Fab' or single chain Fv (scFv) molecules since they do not require the presence of the Fc region for triggering the effector functions of the intact molecule. ScFv are single polypeptide chains made of one heavy chain variable region (VH) linked through a flexible spacer to one light chain variable region (VL) that can be readily cloned and expressed. Second, the exquisite specificity of intact antibodies is maintained, minimising therefore the risk of cross-reactivity with other cellular molecules. In addition, intracellular antibodies, or intrabodies, can be addressed to any cell compartment by adding appropriate localisation sequences by molecular engineering (Fig. 9.1). It allows to stabilise the intrabody and to potentiate its functional effect by increasing its local concentration in the vicinity of the targeted molecule (Cochet *et al.*, 1998a). A recent study by Nizak *et al.* (2003) has shown that intrabodies represent also remarkable conformation sensors and can be used to bind and track specific conformers within a cell, suggesting that they represent indeed a powerful tool both for basic science and therapy.

Intrabodies have been used against a number of molecules with various sub-cellular localisations (Fig. 9.1). They have provided the basis for phenotypic knock-outs («Antibody-Mediated Knock-Out», AMKO) via the binding and sometimes the relocalisation of the targeted antigen. Besides their use to neutralise molecules or block antigen-trafficking within cells, intrabodies have been also used to restore biological functions such as transcriptional activity. The first intrabody to be reported was a recombinant Fab' directed against the gp160 HIV-1 protein (Marasco *et al.*, 1993), present in the endoplasmic reticulum (ER). Intrabodies have been also targeted to oncogenic molecules bound to the inner face of the plasma membrane (p21^ras) (Cochet *et al.*, 1998b; Tanaka and Rabbitts, 2003) or present in the nucleus (the E7 protein, encoded by the human papilloma virus type 16) (Wang-Johanning *et al.*, 1998). Intrabodies that restore the phenotypic function of mutated p53 tumour suppressor gene products (Caron de Fromentel *et al.*, 1999), or prevent the expression of the high affinity IL-2 receptor on cell surface have been reported (Richardson *et al.*, 1995). Other intrabodies directed against the Syk kinase (Dauvillier *et al.*, 2002), the caspases 3 and 7 (Rajpal and Turi, 2001; Zhu *et al.*, 1999), and the hCyclinT1 (Bai *et al.*, 2003) have been shown to interfere with the functions of these molecules. In addition, it has been reported that intrabodies counteract *in situ* huntingtin aggregation in a cellular model of Huntington's disease (HD). It suggests that intrabody-mediated modulation of abnormal neuronal proteins may contribute to the treatment of neuro-degenerative diseases such as HD, Alzheimer's, Parkinson's, prion disease, and the spino-cerebellar ataxias (Lecerf *et al.*, 2001).

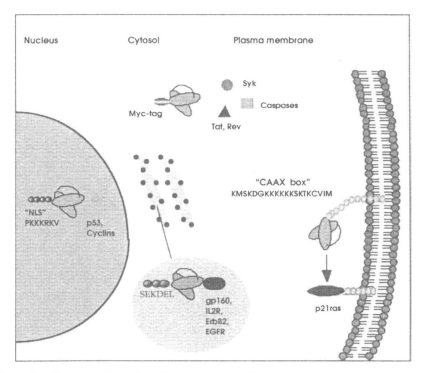

Figure 9.1. Targeting single-chain Fv towards sub-cellular compartments. The addition of localisation (Nuclear Localisation Signal or NLS, CAAX box) or retention (SEKDEL) signals by molecular engineering allows the increase of the antibody concentration in the vicinity of the targeted molecule, thus potentiating the functional effect of the scFv.

Recombinant proteins can be also expressed on the surface of target cells rather than within the cells. In that case, the aim is to recruit and activate immune cells, not to trigger endogenous deleterious events in the targeted cells or to restore a wild-type phenotype. Tumour cells expressing cytokines (Gansbacher *et al.*, 1990; Guarini *et al.*, 1995), MHC class II molecules (Armstrong *et al.*, 1997), co-stimulatory molecules (Townsend and Allison, 1993; Imro *et al.*, 1998), or a combination of these molecules (Hurwitz *et al.*, 1998) have been used to induce tumour regression in mice. Tumour cells have been also engineered to express scFv directed against activating receptors expressed on different cell types of the immune system (Kontermann and Muller, 1999; Gruel *et al.*, 2001). Such antibodies have been termed extrabodies. This approach is particularly attractive when compared to antibodies that target surface antigens: the use of antibodies or bispecific antibodies in cancer therapy requires the generation of anti-tumour antibodies specific for a given tumour type, which has strongly limited the use of therapeutic antibodies in cancer patients so far. Moreover, the injection of antibodies into the peripheral blood of patients has a limited efficacy due to a non-specific binding of the antibodies to $Fc\gamma R^+$ circulating cells and a rapid catabolism.

We describe below in more details the use of intrabodies that interfere with $p21^{ras}$ and p53 functions as well as the expression of an anti-FcγR scFv on the surface of tumour cells to activate immune $Fc\gamma R^+$ cells.

2.   GENERATION AND USE OF INTRABODIES: THE P21RAS AND P53 CASES

An attractive strategy for generating intrabodies is to derive antibody fragments from well-characterised mouse or rat hybridomas. Many well-characterised murine monoclonal antibodies directed against oncogenic or viral molecules are available. However, once a scFv has been cloned and transferred into an eukaryotic expression vector, its expression in mammalian cells under native form can be difficult to obtain. Antibody fragments expressed in the cytosol can be highly aggregated, which reduces their half-life and, thus, their efficacy (Cochet *et al.*, 1998a; Cardinale *et al.*, 2001). This is likely due, at least in part, to the reduced state of scFv present in the reducing environment of the cytosol. Moreover, the monomeric or divalent forms, the levels of expression, and the cellular localisation have also an impact on the functional efficacy of intrabodies. To overcome the problems of misfolding and unstability, a number of approaches have been proposed. First, a selection assay for functional intracellular antibodies using an in-cell two-hybrid system has been described (Visintin *et al.*, 1999). It allows the *de novo* selection of intrabodies from scFv libraries in the reducing environment of yeast. In addition, a common signature of conserved amino-acid residues has been deduced from sequence analysis of scFv isolated using this assay, suggesting that a consensus sequence for intracellular antibodies may characterise stable intrabodies (Visintin *et al.*, 2002). Second, stable and functional scFv without disulfide bonds can be obtained by molecular evolution (Proba *et al.*, 1998) or rational design (Wirtz and Steipe, 1999).

In most cases, the antibody fragment, either Fab' or scFv, exhibits properties similar to the parental antibody, with the same affinity or a decreased affinity. Once cloned, the versatility of recombinant antibody fragments for intracellular targeting is remarkable. The N-Terminus or the C-Terminus part of scFvs can be fused to sequences that allow to target various cell compartments (Fig. 9.1). SEKDEL sequence allows the retention of recombinant antibodies within the ER and, hence, can be used to block the expression of receptors on the cell surface (Richardson *et al.*, 1995; Bilbao *et al.*, 2002) or the assembly of virions (Marasco *et al.*, 1993).

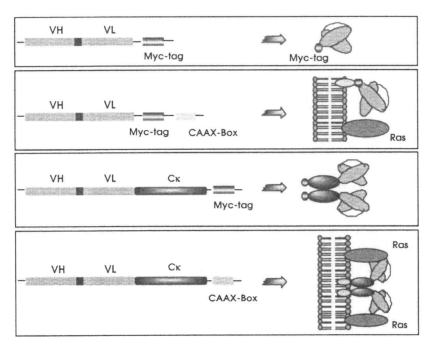

Figure 9.2. The addition of a CAAX box localisation signal sequence (upper middle panel) or of a Cκ sequence derived from the human κ light chain (lower middle panel), or both (lower panel), at the 3' of an anti-Ras cDNA scFv increases the stability and potentiate the neutralisation of mutated Ras (Cochet *et al.*, 1998a ; Cochet *et al.*, 1998b).

The Nuclear Localisation Signal (NLS) sequence derived from the SV40 T antigen makes it possible to target nuclear proteins such as p53, although the latter molecule has been shown to induce the translocation of anti-p53 scFvs lacking NLS signal (Caron de Fromentel *et al.*, 1999). The CAAX box motif can be used to target molecules present at the inner face of plasma membrane. Its addition to the anti-Ras Y13-259 scFv allowed to increase the scFv half-life and its neutralising effect (Cochet *et al.*, 1998a) (Fig. 9.2). Similarly, the addition of the constant domain of the human Cκ light chain at the C-terminus part of the scFv (Fig. 9.2) allows to improve significantly the stability of recombinant antibody fragments (Cochet *et al.*, 1998a; Mhashilkar *et al.*, 1995). It is likely due to the ability of Cκ regions to form homodimers. These dimers exhibit an increased avidity for the antigen due to their divalent structure, which provokes a stronger antibody/antigen interaction, thus stabilising the scFv molecule. This approach has been proved useful for stabilising the anti-Ras Y13-259 scFv (Cochet *et al.*, 1998a). Interestingly, the cytosolic distribution of the anti-Ras scFv-Cκ was found identical to the unmodified anti-Ras scFv. However, the fusion molecule was detected for much longer periods of time in transfected cells. However, the addition of the Cκ domain did not significantly improve the neutralising efficacy of the scFv. Only, the anti-Ras Y13-259 scFv-CAAX or the anti-Ras Y13-259 scFv-Cκ-CAAX exhibited an increase ability to inhibit Ras-induced signalling and to induce apoptosis. Thus, the concentration of scFv in the vicinity of the target molecule can markedly increase its stability and efficacy, even when it shows a tendency to aggregate when expressed as an unmodified form in the cytosol. The ability of scFv to readily interact with the target molecule is a critical parameter to ensure its stability and efficacy as shown by experiments performed with anti-p53 scFv (Caron de Fromentel *et al.*, 1999). When two anti-p53 scFv were expressed in tumour cells, their localisation was dependent on the presence or absence of p53 in the cells. ScFv were detected in the nuclei of tumour cells expressing p53, even in absence of a NLS sequence at their C-terminus end, indicating that the p53-scFv complexes are translocated into the nucleus by the signalling nuclear sequence of p53. By contrast, when the unmodified scFv were expressed in p53$^{-/-}$ cells, they exhibited only a cytosolic localisation, with a patchy aspect.

The function of the anti-ras Y13-259 scFv was investigated by studying its effect on the transcription from the polyoma virus-thymidine kinase (Py-TK) promoter that is strongly activated by expression of Ras in NIH 3T3 cells. Cells were co-transfected with a plasmid containing the chloramphenicol acetyl transferase (CAT) gene under the control of the Py-TK promoter, and expression vectors containing an oncogenic Ras and the Y13-259 scFv under the control of the SV40 early promoter. Oncogenic Ras strongly enhanced the rate of transcription from the Py element. Expression of Y13-259 scFv inhibited activation of the Ras-responsive element that resulted from the expression of Ras. To further demonstrate the specificity of Y13-259 scFv effect, whether the scFv would affect oncogenic Raf transcriptional activity, which is independent from cellular Ras, was studied. The transcriptional activation of the Ras-reporter gene induced by oncogenic Raf was not inhibited by expression of Y13-259 scFv. Finally, a control scFv, derived from the non-neutralising anti-ras Y13-238 antibody (Cochet *et al.*, 1998c), had no effect on either Ras or Raf-induced CAT activity. Apoptosis was then examined by monitoring the percent viability of *in vitro* cultured HCT116, a colon carcinoma cell line expressing a mutant Ki-Ras gene, injected with either Y13-259 or Y13-238 scFv plasmids. In contrast to cells injected with control scFv plasmid, only a small percentage of HCT116 cells injected with Y13-259 scFv was still viable after one day in culture. This loss of viability was shown to occur via an apoptotic pathway as measured by DNA end-labelling techniques. *In vivo* experiments using the anti-Ras Y13-259 scFv strengthened these observations and have been promising on a clinical point of view. The Y13-259 scFv cDNA was cloned into an adenoviral vector, downstream of a CMV promoter. The injection of a single dose of 2×10^9 pfu of Ad-Y13-259 scFv into pre-established HCT116 tumours dramatically affected tumour growth which was efficiently stopped for 20 days. However, tumour growth resumed after that period. When multiple injections of the same dose of Y13-259-expressing adenovirus were realised, tumour regression was much more pronounced and the animals remained tumour-free for an additional 20 days (Cochet *et al.*, 1998b). The capacity of intrabodies to act *in vivo* as therapeutic molecules has been also demonstrated in other models (Curiel, 2000).

The *in vitro* functional efficacy of intrabodies has been also exemplified using anti-p53 intracellular antibodies (Caron de Fromentel *et al.*, 1999). In that case, the aim was not to neutralise the mutated molecule but to restore its transactivating activity. Some anti-p53 monoclonal antibodies are able to increase the sequence-specific DNA binding of wild-type (wt) p53 and to restore the sequence-specific DNA binding of some p53 mutants *in vitro* (Hupp *et al.*, 1992). Anti-p53 scFvs were derived from two of these antibodies and tested for their ability to induce a phenotypic reversion. They were first tested for their ability to enhance the DNA binding activity of wt p53 or to restore the DNA binding activity of p53 mutant His273, by electrophoretic mobility shift assay. Both scFvs were able to enhance or restore the DNA binding of wt or mutant p53, respectively. One scFv was then cloned into an eukaryotic expression vector. Another construct was also derived, in which the nuclear localisation signal (NLS) from SV40 large T antigen was added at the C-terminus of the scFv. When the p53$^{-/-}$ H1299 human lung carcinoma cell line was transfected with the scFv cDNA alone, cytoplasmic staining and possibly nuclear staining were detectable, showing that the scFv was stably expressed in the cells. The co-expression of the mutant p53 His273 strongly increased the concentration of the scFv in the nucleus, even in absence of the NLS sequence, suggesting that p53 and the scFv were able to associate in cells and that p53 was able to drive the scFv into the nucleus. The ability of the scFv to restore the DNA binding activity and the transcriptional function of p53 mutants was then examined. The tumour cell line H1299 was co-transfected with various combinations of plasmids encoding the CAT reporter gene under the control of a p53 responsive element, the scFv, wt p53, p53 mutant His273 or His175. The expression of the scFv, scFv-NLS or the p53 mutant His175 did not affect the basal level of CAT activity. The expression of the p53 mutant His273 led to a weak transcriptional activity, corresponding to 10% of the signal obtained with wt p53. Co-expression of the scFv or scFv-NLS with the p53 mutant His273 led to an increase in the His273-associated transcriptional activity. This effect was not observed with the His175 mutant which had previously been shown to be unsensitive to the activation induced by the antibody used to derived the scFv (Hupp *et al.*, 1993). Thus, this work is an interesting example where intrabodies can supply a gain of function, *i.e.,* the restoration of the deficient transactivating function of a nuclear transcription factor, besides being used as neutralising molecules.

3.   EXTRABODIES ON TUMOUR CELLS: RECRUITING IMMUNE CELLS

The use of extrabodies has been first described to re-direct T cell cytotoxicity (Hwu *et al.*, 1995). Chimeric antibody/T-cell receptor genes composed of the variable domains from monoclonal antibodies joined to T-cell receptor-signalling chains were designed. It was then demonstrated that T cells retrovirally transduced with these genes, termed T-bodies, can recognise antibody-defined antigens and that this recognition leads to T-cell activation, specific lysis, and cytokine release. Conversely, one can think that recombinant antibodies expressed on tumour cells and directed against activating molecules on immune cells could act as a trigger to induce a reverse cytotoxicity and other effects (the «Hooking tumour strategy»). Ideally, the targeted antigen should be expressed on a variety of immune cells harbouring different effector functions, by contrast to the T-bodies that are restricted to a small subset of cytotoxic T cells. An interesting target candidate is FcR. The targeting of FcγR or FcαR by a specific ligand expressed on tumour cells has multiple advantages compared to the surface expression of other proteins such as CD3 or co-stimulatory molecules. In contrast to these molecules, FcR are widely expressed on a large variety of

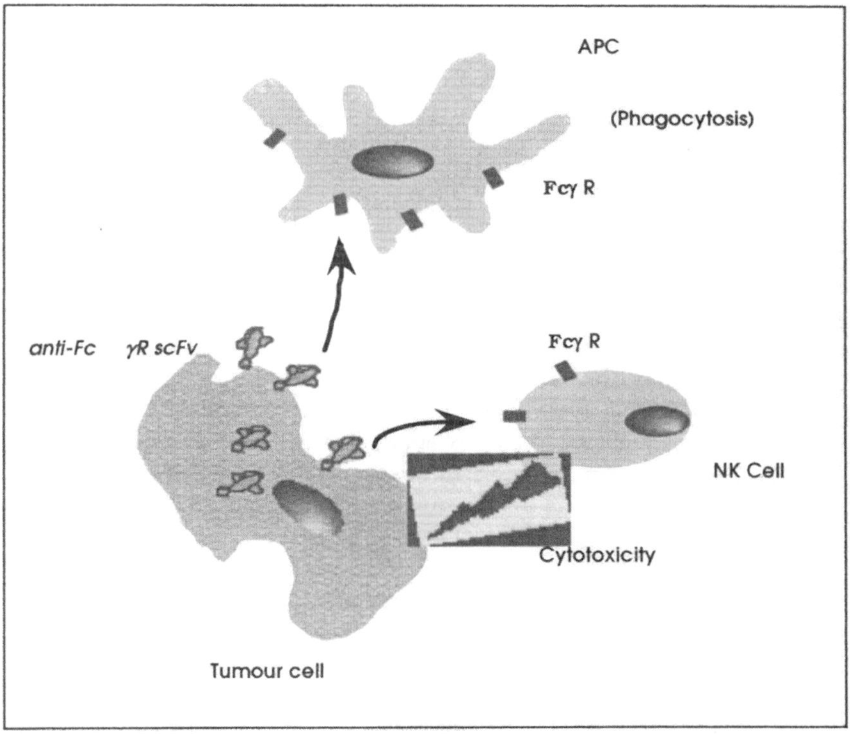

Figure 9.3. Immunotherapy strategy based on the expression of anti-FcγR scFv on tumour cells (the «Hooking tumour strategy»). FcγR⁺ NK cells can be recruited to kill tumour cells through the activation of FcγRIII. The enhancement of phagocytosis of tumour cells or cell extracts by antigen-presenting cells through FcγR could also induce a protective long-term immunity to tumours by allowing recruitment of specific T cells.

cells of the immune system and their engagement provokes the activation of multiple cell functions (Hulett and Hogarth, 1994). Interestingly, cells from both innate and adaptative immunity can be recruited and activated by the binding to and triggering of FcR. On the one hand, potent FcγR⁺ killer cells such as G-CSF-activated neutrophils or NK cells can be recruited to directly kill tumour cells through the activation of FcγRI (Michon *et al.*, 1995) or FcγRIII (Weiner *et al.,* 1993), respectively. On the other hand, the enhancement of phagocytosis of tumour cells or cell extracts by antigen-presenting cells such as dendritic cells through FcγR could induce a protective long-term immunity to tumours by allowing recruitment of T cells

(Kalergis and Ravetch, 2002). An approach based on the expression of anti-FcγR scFv on tumour cells was therefore developed. The ability of tumour-expressed anti-FcγR scFv to activate immune cells *in vitro* and to prevent tumour growth *in vivo* was then examined (Gruel *et al.*, 2001) (Fig. 9.3).

A functional scFv directed against human FcγRIII (CD16) was derived from the 3G8 mouse monoclonal antibody and fused to the transmembrane domain of the Platelet-Derived Growth Factor Receptor (PDGF-R). The scFv was then expressed at the surface of human H1299 lung carcinoma cells. Its binding to soluble biotinylated FcγRIII ectodomains indicated that the fusion molecule was correctly folded and expressed at the tumour cell surface. It induced the secretion of IL-2 and TNFα when tumour cells were co-cultured with FcγRIII$^+$ transfected T cells (Jurkat-CD16/γ) or monocytes, respectively. Furthermore, NK cells killed HLA$^+$ class I H1299 lung carcinoma tumour cells expressing the anti-FcγRIII scFv but not the parental cells, indicating that the expression of anti-FcγRIII scFv at the tumour cell surface can overcome the Killer Inhibitory Receptor (KIR)-mediated inhibition of NK cell cytotoxicity. The presence of anti-FcγRIII scFv on H1299 cells also enhanced tumour phagocytosis by FcγR$^+$ antigen-presenting cells. Last, *in vivo* Winn tests performed in SCID mice indicated that the expression of anti-CD16 scFv at the tumour cell surface prevents the growth of H1299 cells.

The recruitment of effector immune cells by anti-FcγR scFv expressed on the surface of tumour cells has a number of advantages. First, it allows to trigger FcγR-dependent cell functions and to induce cell cytotoxicity without requiring the isolation and use of specific anti-tumour antibodies. This represents an important benefit since many tumours do not express specific tumour antigens and only a few monoclonal antibodies that can be used to target cancer cells are available. Second, the negative immuno-modulatory function exerted by KIR on NK cells can be prevented by expressing anti-FcγRIII antibodies on HLA$^+$ tumour cells otherwise resistant to NK cell activity. The balance between the positive signal triggered by FcγRIII and the negative signal due to the KIR/HLA interaction can be modified in favour of the cytotoxic pathway.

Thus, anti-FcγRIII scFv expressed on tumour cells may be a useful therapeutic tool, since it has been suggested that KIR are responsible for the lack of control of tumour cell growth by killer cells (Mingari *et al.*, 1998). It has also several advantages over the use of engineered bispecific antibodies directed against FcγR and tumour antigens (Segal *et al.*, 1999). No systemic delivery is needed: an intra-tumour gene delivery system can be used, allowing the expression of the anti-FcγR scFv *in situ*. It will avoid the rapid clearance of the injected antibody by FcγR$^+$ cells present in the peripheral blood.

4.   CONCLUSIONS

Although the use of intrabodies represents an exciting approach to treat patients with diseases where no drugs are available, there are still a number of important problems that are likely to hamper its success. First, an adequate delivery of the cDNA encoding the antibody fragment into the targeted cells remains elusive, as methods for *in vivo* gene delivery are still poorly controlled. The extrabody approach described above may represent a peculiar case. One can expect that the recruitment of even a limited number of FcγR⁺ cells can be sufficient to trigger a potent anti-tumour immune response, although it has still to be documented in animal models. Second, the cloning and the expression of functional intrabodies is far from being trivial. Although the generation of scFvs from hybridomas can be readily performed in many cases, the cloning of functional variable regions can be made difficult due to : i) a lack of amplification of VH or VL cDNA even when using primers optimised for RT-PCR and/or ii) the presence of aberrant variable region transcripts which are preferentially amplified. In addition, the lack of clearly defined structural rules that are predictive of intrabody stability makes it difficult to generate the most efficient intracellular antibodies so far. Progress in the knowledge of antibody fragment stability and in techniques for screening thermodynamically optimised scFv will make available a new generation of intrabodies. The emergence of this new wave of antibodies, that are naturally "rationally designed" by the immune system to bind antigens with high specificity and affinity, is an exciting and promising new. There is no doubt that intrabodies will be used in the future as intracellular drugs with exquisite specificity and the remarkable capacity of a fine tuning of the targeted molecules, once gene delivery technologies will have come to an age of maturity.

ACKNOWLEDGEMENTS

We would like to thank all our colleagues who participated in our work on intrabodies over the last decade. We also thank Pr. W.H. Fridman for constant support.

REFERENCES

Armstrong, T.D., Clements, V.K., Martin, B.K., Ting, J.P., and Ostrand-Rosenberg, S., 1997, Major histocompatibility complex class II-transfected tumor cells present endogenous antigen and are potent inducers of tumor-specific immunity. *Proc. Natl. Acad. Sci. USA* **94**: 6886-6891

Bai, J., Sui, J., Zhu, R.Y., Tallarico, A.S., Gennari, F., Zhang, D., and Marasco, W.A., 2003, Inhibition of Tat-mediated transactivation and HIV-1 replication by human anti-hCyclinT1 intrabodies. *J. Biol. Chem.* **278**: 1433-1442

Bilbao, G., Contreras, J.L., and Curiel, D.T., 2002, Genetically engineered intracellular single-chain antibodies in gene therapy. *Mol. Biotechnol.* **22**: 191-211

Biocca, S., Neuberger, M.S., and Cattaneo, A., 1990, Expression and targeting of intracellular antibodies in mammalian cells. *The EMBO J.* **9**: 101-108

Cardinale, A., Filesi, I., and Biocca, S., 2001, Aggresome formation by anti-Ras intracellular scFv fragments. The fate of the antigen-antibody complex. *Eur. J. Biochem.* **268**: 268-277

Caron de Fromentel, C., Gruel, N., Venot, C., Debussche, L., Conseiller, E., Dureuil, C., Teillaud, J.-L., Tocqué, B., and Bracco, L., Restoration of transcriptional activity of p53 mutants in human tumor cells by intracellular expression of anti-p53 single chain Fv fragments. *Oncogene,* 1999, **18**: 551-557

Cochet, O., Delumeau, I., Kenigsberg, M., Gruel, N., Schweighoffer, F., Bracco, L., Teillaud, J.-L., and Tocqué, B., 1998a, Intracellular targeting of oncogenes: a novel approach for cancer therapy. In *Intrabodies* (W.A. Marasco, ed.), Landes R.G. Company, Chapman & Hall, New York, pp.129-142

Cochet, O., Kenigsberg, M., Delumeau, I., Virone-Oddos, A., Multon, M.-C., Fridman, W.H., Schweighoffer, F., Teillaud, J.-L., and Tocqué, B., 1998b, Intracellular expression of an antibody fragment neutralizing p21^{ras} promotes tumor regression. *Cancer Res.* **58**: 1170-1176

Cochet, O., Kenigsberg, M., Delumeau, I., Duchesne, M., Schweighoffer, F., Tocqué, B., and Teillaud, J.-L., 1998c, Intracellular expression and functional properties of an anti-p21^{ras} scFv derived from a rat hybridoma containing specific λ and irrelevant κ light chains. *Mol. Immunol.* **35**: 1097-1110

Cohen, P.A., 2002, Intrabodies. Targeting scFv expression to eukaryotic intracellular compartments. *Methods Mol. Biol.* **178**: 367-378

Curiel, D.T., 2000, Gene therapy for carcinoma of the breast: genetic ablation strategies. *Breast Cancer Res.* **2**: 45-49

Dauvillier, S., Merida, P., Visintin, M., Cattaneo, A., Bonnerot, C., and Dariavach, P., 2002, Intracellular single-chain variable fragments directed to the Src homology 2 domains of Syk partially inhibit FcεRI signaling in the RBL-2H3 cell line. *J. Immunol.* **169**: 2274-2283

Gansbacher, B., Bannerji, R., Daniels, B., Zier, K., Cronin, K., and Gilboa, E., 1990, Retroviral vector-mediated γ-interferon gene transfer into tumor cells generates potent and long lasting anti-tumor immunity. *Cancer Res.* **50**: 7820-7825

Gruel, N., Fridman, W.H., and Teillaud, J.-L., 2001, By-passing tumor-specific and bispecific antibodies: triggering antitumor immunity by expression of anti-FcγR scFv on cancer cell surface. *Gene Therapy* **8**: 1721-1728

Guarini, A., Gansbacher, B., Cronin, K., Fierro, M.T., and Foa, R., 1995, IL-2 gene-transduced human HLA-A2 melanoma cells can generate a specific anti-tumor cytotoxic T-lymphocyte response. *Cytokines & Mol. Ther.* **1**: 57-64

Hulett, M.D., and Hogarth, P.M., 1994, Molecular basis of Fc receptor function. *Adv. Immunol.* **57**: 1-127

Hupp, T.R., Meek, D.W., Midgley, C.A., Lane, D.P., 1992, Regulation of the specific DNA binding function of p53. *Cell* **71**: 875-886

Hupp, T.R., Meek, D.W., Midgley, C.A., Lane, D.P., 1993, Activation of the cryptic DNA binding function of mutant forms of p53. *Nucleic Acids Res.* **21**: 3167-3174

Hurwitz, A.A., Townsend, S.E., Yu, T.F., Wallin, J.A., and Allison, J.P., 1998, Enhancement of the anti-tumor immune response using a combination of interferon-γ and B7 expression in an experimental mammary carcinoma. *Int. J. Cancer* **77**: 107-113

Hwu, P., Yang, J.C., Cowherd, R., Treisman, J., Shafer, G.E., Eshhar, Z., and Rosenberg, S.A., 1995, In vivo antitumor activity of T cells redirected with chimeric antibody/T-cell receptor genes. *Cancer Res.* **55**: 3369-3373

Imro, M.A., Dellabona, P., Manici, S., Heltai, S., Consogno, G., Bellone, M., Rugarli, C., and Protti, M.P., 1998, Human melanoma cells transfected with the B7-2 co-stimulatory molecule induce tumor-specific CD8+ cytotoxic T lymphocytes *in vitro*. *Human Gene Ther.* **9**: 1335-1344

Kalergis, A.M., and Ravetch, J.V., 2002, Inducing tumor immunity through the selective engagement of activating Fcγ receptors on dendritic cells. *J. Exp. Med.* **195**: 1653-1659

Kontermann, R.E., and Muller, R. 1999, Intracellular and cell surface displayed single-chain diabodies. *J. Immunol. Methods* **22**: 179-188

Lecerf, J.M., Shirley, T.L., Zhu, Q., Kazantsev, A., Amersdorfer, P., Housman, D.E., Messer, A., and Huston, J.S., 2001, Human single-chain Fv intrabodies counteract *in situ* huntingtin aggregation in cellular models of Huntington's disease. *Proc. Natl. Acad. Sci. USA* **98**: 4764-4769

Marasco, W.A., Haseltine, W.A., and Chen, S.Y., 1993, Design, intracellular expression, and activity of a human anti-human immunodeficiency virus type 1 gp120 single-chain antibody. *Proc. Natl. Acad. Sci. USA* **90**: 7427-7429

Marasco, W.A., 2001, Intrabodies as antiviral agents. *Curr. Top. Microbiol. Immunol.* **260**: 247-270

Mehren, Mv.M., Adams, G.P., and Weiner, L.M., 2003, Monoclonal antibody therapy for cancer. *Annu. Rev. Med.* **54**: 343-369

Mhashilkar, A.M., Bagley, J., Chen, S.Y., Szilvay, A.M., Helland, D.G., Marasco, W.A., 1995, Inhibition of HIV-1 Tat-mediated LTR transactivation and HIV-1 infection by anti-Tat single chain intrabodies. *EMBO J.* **14**: 1542-1551

Michon, J., Moutel, S., Barbet, J., Romet-Lemonne, J.-L., Deo, Y.M., Fridman, W.H., Teillaud, J.-L., 1995, *In vitro* killing of neuroblastoma cells by neutrophils derived from granulocyte colony-stimulating factor-treated cancer patients using an anti-disialoganglioside/anti-FcγRI bispecific antibody. *Blood* **86**: 1124-1130

Mingari, M.C., Moretta, A., Moretta, L., 1998, Regulation of KIR expression in human T cells: a safety mechanism that may impair protective T-cell responses. *Immunol. Today* **19**: 153-157

Nizak, C., Monier, S., del Nery, E., Moutel, S., Goud, B., and Perez, F., 2003, Recombinant antibodies to the small GTPase Rab6 as conformation sensors. *Science* **300**: 984-987

Proba, K., Worn, A., Honegger, A., and Plückthun, A., 1998, Antibody scFv fragments without disulfide bonds made by molecular evolution. *J. Mol. Biol.* **275**: 245-253

Rajpal, A., and Turi, T.G., 2001, Intracellular stability of anti-caspase-3 intrabodies determines efficacy in retargeting the antigen. *J. Biol. Chem.* **276**: 33139-33146

Richardson, J.H., Sodroski, J.G., Waldmann, T.A., and Marasco, W.A., 1995, Phenotypic knockout of the high-affinity human interleukin 2 receptor by intracellular single-chain antibodies against the alpha sub-unit of the receptor. *Proc. Natl. Acad. Sci. USA* **92**: 3137-3141

Segal, D.M., Weiner, G.J., Weiner, L.M., 1999, Bispecific antibodies in cancer therapy. *Cur. Opinion in Immunol.* **11**: 558-562

Tanaka, T, and Rabbitts, T.H., 2003, Intrabodies based on intracellular capture frameworks that bind the RAS protein with high affinity and impair oncogenic transformation. *EMBO J.* **22**: 1025-1035

Townsend, S.E., and Allison, J.P., 1993, Tumor rejection after direct co-stimulation of CD8+ T cells by B7-transfected melanoma cells. *Science* **259**: 368-370

Visintin, M., Tse, E., Axelson, H., Rabbitts, T.H., and Cattaneo, A., 1999, Selection of antibodies for intracellular function using a two-hybrid *in vivo* system. *Proc. Natl. Acad. Sci. USA* **9**: 11723-11728

Visintin, M., Settanni, G., Maritan, A., Graziosi, S., Marks, J.D., and Cattaneo, A., 2002, The intracellular antibody capture technology (IACT): towards a consensus sequence for intracellular antibodies. *J. Mol. Biol.* **317**: 73-83

Wang-Johanning, F., Gillespie, G.Y., Grim., J., Rancourt, C., Alvarez, R.D., Siegal, G.P., and Curiel, D.T., 1998, Intracellular expression of a single-chain antibody directed against human papillomavirus type 16 E7 oncoprotein achieves targeted antineoplastic effects. *Cancer Res.* **58**: 1893-1900

Wirtz, P., and Steipe, B., 1999, Intrabody construction and expression III: engineering hyperstable V(H) domains. *Protein Sci.* **8**: 2245-2250

Weiner, L.M., Holmes, M., Adams, G.P., LaCreta, F., Watts, P., and Garcia de Palazzo, I., 1993, A human tumor xenograft model of therapy with a bispecific monoclonal antibody targeting c-erbB-2 and CD16. *Cancer Res.* **53**: 94-100

Zhu, Q., Zeng, C., Huhalov, A., Yao, J., Turi, T.G., Danley, D., Hynes, T., Cong, Y., DiMattia, D., Kennedy, S., Daumy, G., Schaeffer, E., Marasco, W.A., and Huston, J.S., 1999, Extended half-life and elevated steady-state level of a single-chain Fv intrabody are critical for specific intracellular retargeting of its antigen, caspase-7. *J. Immunol. Methods* **231**: 207-22.

Chapter 10

ANTITUMOR ANTIBODIES: FROM RESEARCH TO CLINIC

Sylvie Ménard, Serenella M. Pupa, Manuela Campiglio and Elda Tagliabue
Molecular Targeting Unit, Dept. of Experimental Oncology, Istituto Nazionale Tumori, Milan, Italy, Bioeurope 2001, European Conference on Biopharmaceutical Antibodies, Como, 20-22 Giugno 2001

Over the last 15 years, we have produced monoclonal antibodies directed specifically against tumor cells, especially carcinoma cells. 150.000 supernatants of growing hybridoma cells coming from 150 different somatic fusions of spleen cells from mice immunized with different immunogens and protocols, were screened for specific reactivity on tumor cells. Only 45 monoclonal antibodies were selected for basic researches and clinical applications.

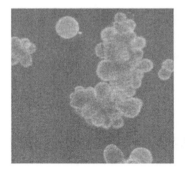

Figure 10.1. Immunoreactivity of a pool of MAbs on breast tumor cells from pleuric effusion.

The majority of the immunizations were performed using tumor extracts or tumor cells derived from carcinoma surgical specimens. Screening of antibodies was performed by immunofluorescence, immunohistochemical or binding tests. The first category of monoclonal antibodies was selected for diagnosis and prognosis. They mainly include reagents directed against epithelial cells, that when used as a pool, are able to recognize 100% of breast carcinomas and to discriminate e.g. the breast histotype from the ovary carcinomas (Ménard et al., 1994; Tagliabue et al., 1986) (Figure 10.1). The second category includes antibodies recognizing adhesion molecules receptors, proteolytic enzymes or growth factors receptors which are often overexpressed in tumor cells (Figure 10.2) and therefore were found to discriminate tumor from the normal counterpart and to investigate the interactions between tumor and microenviroment. Most of these MAbs have been proved useful for cancer diagnosis and prognosis. Our pool of mono-specific reagents directed against anti-epithelial tumor-associated molecules has been used for the detection of micro metastasis in lymph-nodes and bone marrow, as well as for detection of cancer cells in effusion (Ménard et al., 1994). Some of the antibodies endowed of tissue-specific reactivity can be used for the identification of the source of metastatic lesions. Monoclonal antibodies recognizing molecules with altered expression in tumors can be extremely helpful to draw a biomolecular profile of tumor for either prognostic purposes or for prediction of response to therapy (Ménard et al., 1999).

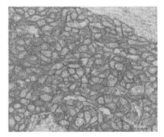

Figure 10.2. Immunoreactivity with an anti-HER2 MAb on breast carcinoma surgical specimens overexpressing the oncoprotein

However, the most important application for monoclonal antibodies is their potential use for anti-tumor therapy. To this aim, the monoclonal antibodies directed against EGF receptor (Baselga et al., 2000; Herbst et al., 2002) or HER2 (Slamon et al., 2001; Vogel et al., 2002) or the folate-receptor (Canevari et al., 1995; van Zanten-Przybysz et al., 2001) have been proved appropriate. An important parameter to select monospecific agents for therapy is the recognized antigenic epitopes, since some antibodies have been found to inhibit or even to stimulate the receptor function according to the determinant recognized. Also the affinity and the avidity of the antibodies condition their therapeutic activity.

All MAbs selected so far display the same range of affinity ($K_{aff}= 10^{-7}-10^{-8}$). Various hypotheses may explain the homogeneity of such parameter as the homology of the recognized target antigen with endogenous protein which in turn restraints the possibility of immune recognition because of elimination of clones with high affinity. Alternatively, the methodology of screening might be particularly adequate for selection of MAbs with this range of affinity.

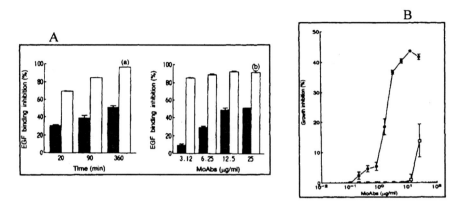

Figure 10.3. A) Inhibition of EGF binding to its receptor by anti-EGFR MAb in its monovalent (empty bar) or bivalent (solid bar) form; B) in vitro growth inhibition of EGF receptor overexpressing carcinoma cell line by anti-EGFR antibody according to its valency. (•) bivalent antibody, (□) monovalent antibody.

Also valency of the MAb plays a relevant role in the therapeutic activity of the reagent. Even if the binding of anti-EGFr MAb on tumor cells is prevalently monovalent, only the bivalent Mab is internalized and inhibits *in vitro* proliferation (Nishikawa et al., 1992).

According to *in vitro* data, also *in vivo* in developed preclinical models, indicate that only the bivalent antibody display a therapeutic activity (Morelli et al., 1994) (Figure 10.3).

In addition, also antibodies directed against drugs, such as doxorubicin, were found useful to modulate drug toxicity. For example, our MAbs directed against doxorubicin were found to inhibit drug-induced alopecia and mucositis (Balsari et al., 1994) (Figure 10.4).

A   B

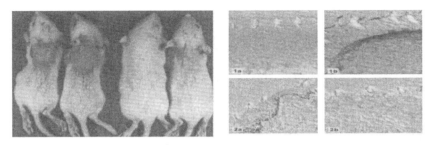

Figure 10.4. A) Head and proximal neck severe alopecia in rats treated with DXR only (left); negative and mild alopecia in rats treated with DXR + anti-DXR MAb (right); B)Parasagittal section of murine tongue illustrating protection from DXR induced apoptosis by anti-DXR MAb. 1a – tongue of untreated animal. 1b – tongue of DXR treated animal, 2a – tongue of DXR treated animal orally treated with unrelated antibody, 2b – tongue of DXR treated animal orally treated with anti-DXR antibody.

The experience of the National Cancer Institute of Milan (Italy) in the treatment of tumor bearing patients based on the use of monoclonal antibodies concerns a MAb directed against the folate receptor which is overexpressed in the majority of ovarian carcinomas. This reagent has been delivered as a hybrid antibody for the retargeting of activated patient's lymphocytes and it has been shown to significantly increase disease-free survival (Canevari et al., 1995). Even antibodies to growth factor receptors (anti-EGFr and HER2) resulted to mediate anti-proliferative properties *in vitro*.

Steering a monoclonal antibody from the laboratory to the clinic/marketplace is a long way. Indeed, good ideas and good antibodies need certain infrastructure and intradisciplinary expertise to turn a positive lab bench result into a successful clinical drug and a viable commercial product.

In conclusions, MAbs are potential therapeutic tools for cancer therapy. Efforts to determine how they work *in vivo* might allow improving their selection, manipulation and the clinic treatment schedule.

REFERENCES

Balsari AL, Morelli D, Ménard S, Veronesi U. Colnaghi MI. 1994. Protection against doxorubicin-induced alopecia in rats by liposome-entrapped monoclonal antibodies. FASEB J 8:226-230.

Baselga J, Pfister D, Cooper MR, Cohen R, Burtness B, Bos M, D'Andrea G, Seidman A, Norton L, Gunnett K, Falcey J, Anderson V, Waksal H, Mendelsohn J. 2000. Phase I studies of anti-epidermal growth factor receptor chimeric antibody C225 alone and in combination with cisplatin. J Clin Oncol 18:904-914.

Canevari S, Stoter G, Arienti F, Bolis G, Colnaghi MI, Di Re E, Eggermont AMM, Goey SH, Gratama JW, Lamers CHJ, Nooy MA, Parmiani G, Raspagliesi F, Ravagnani F, Scarfone G, Trimbos JB, Warnaar SO, Bolhuis RLH. 1995. Regression of advanced ovarian carcinoma by intraperitoneal treatment with autologous T-lymphocytes retargeted by a bispecific monoclonal antibody. J Natl Cancer Inst 87:1463-1469.

Herbst RS, Langer CJ. 2002. Epidermal growth factor receptors as a target for cancer treatment: the emerging role of IMC-C225 in the treatment of lung and head and neck cancers. Semin Oncol 29:27-36.

Ménard S, Casalini P, Tomasic G, Pilotti S, Cascinelli N, Bufalino R, Perrone F, Longhi C, Rilke F, Colnaghi MI. 1999. Pathobiologic identification of two distinct breast carcinoma subsets with diverging clinical behaviors. Breast Cancer Res Treat 55:169-177.

Ménard S, Squicciarini P, Luini A, Sacchini V, Rovini D, Tagliabue E, Veronesi P, Salvadori B, Veronesi U, Colnaghi MI. 1994. Immunodetection of bone marrow micrometastases in breast carcinoma patients and its correlation with primary tumor prognostic features. Br J Cancer 69:1126-1129.

Morelli D, Villa E, Tagliabue E, Perletti L, Villa ML, Ménard S, Balsari A, Colnaghi MI. 1994. Relevance of antibody valency in EGF receptor modulation. Scand J Immunol 39:453-458.

Nishikawa K, Rosenblum MG, Newman RA, Pandita TK, Hittelman WN, Donato NJ. 1992. Resistance of human cervical carcinoma cells to tumor necrosis factor correlates with their increased sensitivity to cisplatin: Evidence of a role for DNA repair and epidermal growth factor receptor. Cancer Res 52:4758-4765.

Slamon DJ, Leyland-Jones B, Shak S, Fuchs H, Paton V, Bajamonde A, Fleming T, Eiermann W, Wolter J, Pegram M, Baselga J, Norton L. 2001. Use of chemotherapy plus a monoclonal antibody against HER2 for metastatic breast cancer that overexpresses HER2. N Engl J Med 344:783-792.

Tagliabue E, Porro G, Barbanti P, Della Torre G, Ménard S, Rilke F, Colnaghi MI. 1986. Improvement of tumor cell detection using a pool of monoclonal antibodies. Hybridoma 5:107-115.

van Zanten-Przybysz I, Molthoff CF, Roos JC, Verheijen RH, van Hof A, Buist MR, Prinssen HM, Den Hollander W, Kenemans P. 2001. Influence of the route of administration on targeting of ovarian cancer with the chimeric monoclonal antibody MOv18: i.v. vs. i.p. Int J Cancer 92:106-114.

Vogel CL, Cobleigh MA, Tripathy D, Gutheil JC, Harris LN, Fehrenbacher L, Slamon DJ, Murphy M, Novotny WF, Burchmore M, Shak S, Stewart SJ, Press M. 2002. Efficacy and safety of trastuzumab as a single agent in first-line treatment of HER2-overexpressing metastatic breast cancer. J Clin Oncol 20:719-726.

Chapter 11

MACROPHAGES FOR IMMUNOTHERAPY
Activated Macrophages plus anti-tumour antibodies in adoptive immunotherapy

Delphine Loirat, Sylvie Jacod, Aurélie Boyer, Fabrice Auzelle, Andrès McAllister, Jean-Pierre Abastado, Jacques Bartholeyns, Didier Prigent
IDM (Immuno Designed Molecule), 172 rue de Charonne 75545 Paris Cedex 11, France

1.   INTRODUCTION

Macrophage efficiently kill and phagocyte tumour cells *in vitro*. To harness the potential therapeutic value of these cells, we have developed a single use Cell Processor able to generate large number of clinical grade Monocyte-derived Activated Killer cells (MAK®). These macrophages were armed with a bispecific antibody (MDX-H210, Medarex Inc., Keler, 1997), recognizing CD64/FcγR1 (on the MAK cell) and the oncoprotein HER-2/neu on tumour cell and present several anti-tumoural effector functions.

MAK have been injected intravenously, intraperitoneally, intravesically in phase II clinical trials to assess the anti-tumour activity.

More than 1000 injections of these cell drugs have been performed and no serious adverse events were reported.

The present study documents the *ex vivo* functionality of armed MAK/cells (tumour binding, tumour lysis, phagocytosis) and the results of a pilot clinical trial in ovarian cancer patients.

Antibodies, Volume 2: Novel Technologies and Therapeutic Use
Edited by G. Subramanian, Kluwer Academic/Plenum Publishers, New York 2004

2.   GENERATION OF CLINICAL GRADE MAK®

Mononuclear cells are collected by apheresis, seeded in defined culture medium in non adherent hydrophobic bags. After 6 days of incubation in presence of GM-CSF in a closed system (MAK® Cell Processor), differentiated macrophages are activated with γ-IFN and then purified by elutriation. This process allows the production of approximately 1×10^9 MAK per apheresis (Boyer *et al*, 1999). The cells are then incubated with purified bispecific antibodies (MDX-H210) before intraperitoneal injection to ovarian cancer patients. The resulting product, the combination of MAK linked to MDX-H210 bispecific antibody, is referred to as OSIDEM®(Fig. 11.1).

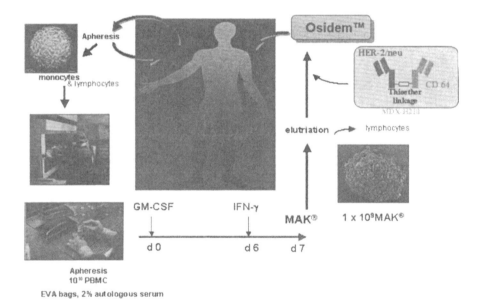

Figure 11.1. OSIDEM® cell drug production scheme for Ovarian Cancer Patient: d0 : day 0 = corresponds to the seeding of mononuclear cells in culture medium containing GM-CSF and autologous serum: d6 : day 6 = corresponds to addition of IFNγ for macrophage activation.

3. EX-VIVO ANTI-TUMOUR FUNCTIONNALITY OF MAK IN THE PRESENCE OR ABSENCE OF BISPECIFIC ANTIBODY MDX-H210.

3.1 Conjugate formation with HER-2/neu positive tumour cells

To assess the targeting of tumour cells by MAK armed with MDX-H210 we have developed an assay that allows detection of conjugates formation between MAK and tumour cells. The target cells used in this assay were SK-OV-3 cell line (HTB 77) derived from human ovarian cancer and over-expressing HER-2/neu tumour antigen. SK-OV-3 cells were stained with PKH-26 membrane dye prior to the assay. MAK armed or not with MDX-H210 were incubated with SK-OV-3 from one to twenty hours at an effector to target ratio of 2:1. Then cells were stained with a CD11c antibody and colocalized events (CD11c positive PKH-26 positive events) were measured by two color flow cytometry (Ely, 1996).

In the presence of antibodies, MAK present significantly increased tumour targeting within one hour, resulting in the formation of MAK-tumour cells conjugates. Moreover, after prolonged incubation (20 hours), clearance of target cells was observed and augmented in the presence of MDX-H210. This activity could be attributed to phagocytosis and/or lysis of SK-OV-3 by MAK, following conjugate formation (Fig. 11.2).

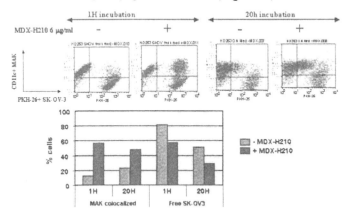

Figure 11.2. OSIDEM™ / SK-OV-3 conjugate-formation assay. Co-incubation of MAK armed with MDX-H210 with SK-OV-3 cells lead to increased clearance of tumour cells,

compared to MAK used without MDX-H210. Top panel: Colocalisation results staining with
fluorescent dyes. Bottom panel : % of conjugated cells with or without MDX-H210

3.2   Antibody dependent cell cytotoxicity

Antibody-dependent cell cytotoxicity (ADCC) was measured in a classical
51-chromium release assay using target cells expressing different levels of
HER-2/neu (Munn et al, 1995, Keller et al 2000). The cells of the M44 cell
line (INSERM U195) derived from a melanoma tumour express low levels
of HER-2/neu on their surface whereas SK-OV-3 (ATCC, HTB 77) and SK-
BR-3 (ATCC, HTB 30) (derived from human breast cancer) overexpress
HER-2/neu antigen. Using this assay we have established that OSIDEM
(MAK cells linked with MDX-H210 bispecific antibody) was able to lyse
target cells overexpressing the HER2/neu antigen (SK-OV-3 and SK-BR-3)
and that lysis was proportional to the expression of HER2/neu. (Fig. 11.3)

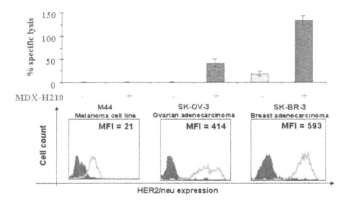

Figure 11.3. In vitro functionality of OSIDEM™ cell drug. ADCC is dependent on HER2/neu
expression on tumour cell lines. Tumour expressing HER2/neu are lysed by MAK linked with
MDX-H210 in the presence of anti-HER2/neu ; the lysis is proportional to HER2/neu
expression level on tumours. Top panel: % of tumour cells lysed by MAK Bottom panel:
intensity of HER2/neu expression by 3 cell lines

3.3   Phagocytosis

To visualize events occurring during the co-incubation of OSIDEM +
SK-OV-3 cells, confocal microscopy was performed (Wallace et al, 2001).
OSIDEM was co-incubated during 4 hours with PKH-26-labeled SK-OV-3.

The incubation was performed either at 4°C or at 37°C, then cells were stained with CD14 specific antibody to distinguish MAK.

At 4°C MAK/SK-OV-3 conjugates could be observed. After incubation at 37°C, most of the MAK present in their cytoplasm some red staining corresponding to SK-OV-3 debris (Fig. 11.4). These results demonstrate that contact between macrophages and tumour cells detected by colocalisation in the presence of anti-tumour antibodies, is followed by phagocytosis of the tumour cells after a 4 hour incubation.

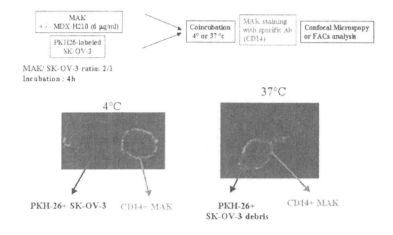

Figure 11.4. MAK armed with MDX-H210 target and phagocyte SK-OV-3 cells. Confocal microscopy of contact between tumour cells and MAK at 4°C and phagocytosis at 37°C.

3.4   Functionality of thawed MAK is preserved

Drug stability is of major importance in product development. While initial clinical trials aimed at establishing the proof of concept were mainly performed with fresh cells, we decided to explore whether MAK cell could be cryopreserved. Such cryopreservation would considerably improve the feasibility and simplify the logistics of MAK-based therapies. To allow preservation of MAK and the injection of multiple doses from a unique cell preparation, we have determined the freezing condition for MAK. MAK were frozen in cryocytes (bags resistant to the freezing process) in 4% Human Serum Albumin, 10 % DMSO at high cell concentration and stored in liquid nitrogen vapor. These conditions allow good cell recovery and viability after thawing.

Thawed MAK were washed and incubated with MDX-H210 antibody and used in functional assays. The functionality of thawed MAK + MDX-H210 was measured by colocalisation assay and ADCC ; both activities were preserved after thawing of cryopreserved MAK (fig. 11.5A and 11.5B). The stability of the cell drugs allows freezing of autologous patient-dedicated lots of MAK to be re-injected sequentially for therapy.

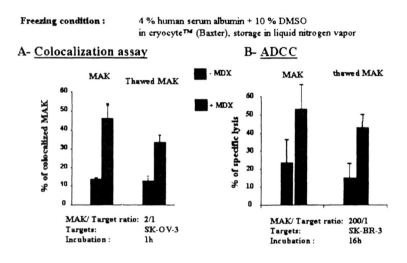

Figure 11.5. Thawed MAK Functionality Left panel: conjugate formation (A) Right panel: ADCC (B)

4.   EFFICACY OF MAK®/MDX-H210 IN CLINICAL STUDY

A Phase I/II clinical trial using OSIDEM™ cell drug (MAK + MDX-H210) was conducted in epithelial ovarian cancer patients, with 6 weekly intra-peritoneal injections of OSIDEM (corresponding to 10^9 MAK cells + MDX-H210). Safety and feasibility of the treatment, as well as signs of clinical activity were demonstrated (de Gramont, 2002).

Study design

14 stage III ovarian cancer patients with microscopic or macroscopic ($\leq$ 1 cm) residual disease after surgery and chemotherapies were included. Patients were treated with one cycle of 6 weekly intra-peritoneal administration of OSIDEM cell drug following 6 apheresis and MAK preparations according to 2-1. (10^9 MAK + 1.5 mg of MDX-H210) :

- In total, 100 MAK cell preparation were administrated during the study
- Only minor adverse events (grade I or II) were observed in a limited number of patients and no serious adverse events related to the product were reported.

Results

3 months evaluation:
In the subgroup who had microscopic lesions before cell therapy, 5 patients had a pathological complete response based on multiple negative biopsies (4 of these patient are alive more than 4 years after treatment). 1 patient showed no change and disease progressed in 2 patients at the time of the third look.

In the patients with macroscopic lesions before treatment, 1 patient had a complete clinical remission, 2 patients showed no change and 3 had developed progressive disease. Interestingly, a significant CA 125 decrease was observed in 2 of these patients.

With a minimum follow-up of 33 months, the one year survival rate was 71 % and 2 year survival was 64 %.

In addition, the safety of intravenous administration of OSIDEM cell drug (MAK + MDX-H210) was assessed in patients with metastatic cancer. The safety and feasibility of 6 weeks IV injections was documented in 10 patients with only minor grade I and II adverse events.

Based on these results and on the good safety profile of OSIDEM, an international multicentre phase III (in Europe, Australia, Canada) trial has been initiated in ovarian carcinoma patients in the consolidation of the clinical response after a second line of chemotherapy.

5.   CONCLUSION

Macrophages are found in the periphery or within tumour tissues. In many instances growing tumours have diverted to their profit the innate immune responses, and these macrophages are rendered tolerogenic or even support angiogenesis allowing tumour spreading. The macrophages that we derive from blood monocytes have not been exposed to the negative tumour signals and have been activated *ex vivo* with gamma interferon to gain specific natural anti-tumoral properties (MAK cells). Among different receptors induced by this activation is the CD64 high affinity type I receptor for IgG. MAK are therefore particularly adequate to fix a bi-specific antibody such as MDX-H210 that binds to FcγRI outside its ligand binding site.

We have shown in *ex vivo* experiments that MAK armed with a bispecific antibody (MDX-H210) recognising HER2/neu on tumour cells and CD64 present a markedly increased anti-tumoural activity as shown by increased phagocytosis as well as lysis of tumours expressing HER2/neu by antibody-dependant cell cytotoxicity. Furthermore, we have shown by co-localisation experiments that the specific targeting of the tumour is enhanced in the presence of the antibodies.

Therefore, MAK have been developed as effector cells which combined with antibodies at very low dose (1.5 mg/10^9 MAK instead of the 100 mg used for direct in vivo antibody therapy) constitute cell drugs prepared according to the principles of good manufacturing practice. These cell drugs can be frozen, kept for several months until thawing before direct re-injection to the patient without losing their effector activity.

Autologous MAK have been prepared in single-use closed systems (cell processors); more than 1000 reproducible and standardized MAK preparations have been manufactured and re-infused to cancer patients. The injections were performed when possible in periphery of the tumour; intra-peritoneally for ovary cancer. The remarkable tolerance of this adoptive anti-tumoural cell immunotherapy should be stressed. No toxicity higher than grade 2 linked to the treatment was reported. This absence of severe adverse events allowed complete preservation of patients quality of life, in contrast to conventional chemotherapy or radiotherapy. The clinical benefits were observed in phase I and II clinical trials in bladder cancer (not presented here) and ovary cancer.

The mechanism of anti-tumoural efficacy of MAK armed with antibodies in cancer patients remains to be clearly demonstrated: there is a direct cytotoxic effect resulting in peripheral tumour necrosis, but delayed actions with anti-tumour effects appearing and lasting for several months or even years are reported. This could suggest the induction of an immune response against tumours which has been documented for dendritic cells but can not be excluded for macrophages.

The very stimulating results achieved in several cancer indications with preservation of quality of life have incited IDM to initiate international multicentre phase III clinical trial with MAK. The clinical results obtained in terms of relapse-free survival and overall survival hopefully will validate this immunotherapy as an alternative anticancer treatment available for a large number of cancer patients in desperate need since not responding to present treatments.

REFERENCES

Boyer A., Andreu G., Romet-Lemonne J.L., Fridman W.H., Teillaud J.L., 1999, Experimental. Haematologyl., **27(4)**: 751-61

De Gramont A., Gangji D., Louvet C., Garcia M.L., Tardy D., Romet-Lemone J.L., 2002, Gynecologic Oncology, **86(1)**: 102,

Ely, 1996, Blood, 87, **238**: 3813-3821

Keler et al, 1997, Cancer Research, **57**: 4008-4014

Keler T., Wallace P.K., Vitale L. A., Russoniello C., Sundarapandiyan K., Graziano R.F., Deo Y. M., 2000, J Immunol, **164**: 5746

Munn D.H., and Cheung N.K., 1995, Cancer Immunology, Immunotherapy, **41**: 46,

Wallace P.K., Kaufman P.A., Lewis L.D., Keler T., Givan A. L., Fisher J. L. , Waugh M. G., Wahner A. E., Guyre P. M., Fanger M. W., Ernstoff M. S., 2001, J Immunol Methods, **248**: 167

Chapter 12

FUTURE PROSPECTS IN ANTIBODY ENGINEERING AND THERAPY

Sophie Siberil[*+], and Jean-Luc Teillaud[*]

[*]Unité INSERM 255, Centre de Recherches Biomédicales des Cordeliers, 15 rue de l'Ecole de Médecine, 75270 Paris cedex 06, France; [+]Laboratoire Français du Fractionnement et des Biotechnologies, Les Ulis, France

1. INTRODUCTION: CURRENT STATUS OF THERAPEUTIC MONOCLONAL ANTIBODIES

Since their discovery by Köhler and Milstein (1975), monoclonal antibodies (mAbs) have been intensively engineered to optimise their therapeutic properties. Although the first mAb to be approved for a clinical use was a murine antibody (OKT3, or Muromomab) (Table 12.1), it became increasingly obvious that only mAbs with a decreased immunogenicity could be used for repeated injections in Humans. The generation of a Human Anti-Mouse Antibody (HAMA) response when murine mAbs are infused to patients hampers their therapeutic efficacy and provokes side-effects related to the formation of immune-complexes. Moreover, studies developed in the 80's indicated that the Fcγ regions of mouse IgG - the most frequent immunoglobulin isotype of mAbs - trigger effector functions in Humans with a lower efficacy than their human Fcγ counterparts. Notably, the level of Complement-Dependent Cytotoxicity (CDC) and of Antibody-Dependent Cell Cytotoxicity (ADCC) that can be achieved is lower when mouse antibodies are used *in vitro* with human serum or cells from human origin, respectively.

Thus, many technical efforts were made to generate a "second generation" of monoclonal antibodies with decreased immunogenicity and optimised effector functions. The development of molecular engineering techniques and a better knowledge of immunoglobulin gene organisation and rearrangements and of immunoglobulin 3-D structure, allowed the engineering of chimeric antibodies (Morrison *et al.*, 1984; Takeda *et al.*, 1985) and of humanized antibodies (Queen *et al.*, 1989; Co and Queen, 1991). A number of these antibodies are now approved and marketed (Table 12.1). However, although these approaches allow the reduction of the immunogenicity of the recombinant molecules, an immune response can be still observed in some patients. The generation of fully human monoclonal antibodies has been therefore a major goal of laboratories involved in mAbs generation since the late 80's and early 90's, even though it is still not clear that such antibodies will have a definitive advantage over these "second generation" chimeric or humanised antibodies. Anti-idiotypic responses could be a problem when using repeatedly fully human monoclonal antibodies at high doses, while the use of chimeric antibodies might divert the human antibody responses against non-critical epitopes, thus preventing neutralisation of the antibody activity.

It has been known for more than two decades that human B lymphocytes can be immortalised following infection with the Epstein-Barr Virus to produce mAbs (Steinitz *et al.*, 1977). However, this technique is limited by serious problems that include selection of antibodies with the desired antigen specificity, cell line stability and yield of antibodies produced for a therapeutic use. Other approaches based on cellular engineering such as the use of molecules inducing a long-term growth of human B lymphocytes or transforming molecules did not proved to be efficient enough or convincingly reproducible to represent a true alternative (Olsson and Kaplan, 1980; Borrebaeck, 1989; Banchereau *et al.*, 1989).

Techniques allowing gene inactivation and insertion of large human DNA fragments from Yeast Artificial Chromosome (YAC) or human chromosome fragments in mouse germline made it possible to generate transgenic mice capable of producing fully human antibodies following immunisation (Lonberg *et al.*, 1994; Green *et al.*, 1994; Tomizuka *et al.*, 2000). Several of these antibodies have been recently used in human clinical trials. Alternatively, the adaptation of the phage display technique (Smith, 1985) to the expression of antibody fragments allowed to build large combinatorial libraries of VH and VL and made it possible to select for specific Fab' or single chain Fv (scFv) fragments (Huse *et al.*, 1989; McCafferty *et al.*, 1990). In addition, phage display is used to generate high-affinity antibody fragments mutated by random or site-directed mutagenesis, thus mimicking the hypermutation process occuring *in vivo* during antibody responses (Hawkins *et al.*, 1992). Although only two of the fourteen mAbs currently approved and marketed (Table 12.1) are fully human antibodies, about 15% of the 140 mAbs currently in clinical development are human antibodies derived either from phage display libraries or from transgenic mice.

Thus, if one compares the current clinical use and forecast of therapeutic antibodies with the situation prevailing less than ten year ago, it is clear that monoclonal antibodies have now come of age as therapeutics.

Table 12.1. Summary of Currently Approved and Marketed Therapeutic mAbs

Antibody	Name	Origin	Molecular target	Indication	Company[§]
OKT3	Orthoclone Muromomab	Mouse	CD3	Transplantation	J&J
Panorex[+]	Edrecolomab	Mouse	EpCAM	Oncology	Centocor, GSK
Reopro	Abciximab	Chimeric	gpIIb/IIIa	CVD[*]	Lilly
Rituxan	Rituximab	Chimeric	CD20	Oncology	Genentech, Roche
Simulect	Basiliximab	Chimeric	CD25	Transplantation	Novartis
Remicade	Infliximab	Chimeric	TNFα	Inflammation	J&J
Zenapax	Daclizumab	Humanised	CD25	Transplantation	Roche
Synagis	Palivizumab	Humanised	RSV[*]	Infectious Disease	Medimmune
Herceptin	Trastuzumab	Humanised	HER2/Neu	Oncology	Genentech, Roche
Mylotarg	Gemtuzumab (Ozogamicin)	Humanised	CD33	Oncology	AHP, Wyeth Lab., Celltech
Campath	Alemtuzumab	Humanised	CD52	Oncology	Millennium
Zevalin	Ibritumomab	^{90}YMouse	CD20	Oncology	IDEC Pharm., Schering AG
Humira	Adalimumab	Human	TNFα	RA[*]	CAT, BASF, Abbott Labs
Enbrel	Etanercept	Human	TNFα	RA[*], PA[*]	Amgen, Immunex

[*]RSV: Respiratory Syncytial Virus; CVD: CardioVascular Diseases/Restenosis; RA: Rheumatoid Arthritis; PA: Psoriatic Arthritis

[+]Approved in Germany not in USA

[§]Marketers/Corporate sponsors

Table 12.2. Summary of mAbs in Phase III Clinical Trials (Oncology)

Antibody	Name	Origin	Molecular target	Indication	Company[§]
Bexxar[+], radiolabeled [131]Iodine	Tositumomab	Mouse	CD20	NHL[*]	Corixa, Coulter Pharmaceuticals, GSK
Erbitux, IMC-C225	Centuximab	Chimeric	EGF-R	CRC[*], head and neck carcinoma	ImClone Systems, BMS
CeaVac		Mouse	Anti-idiotypic, CEA mimic	CRC[*], NSCLC[*]	Titan Pharmaceuticals
Avastin	Bevacizumab	Humanised	VEGF	CRC[*], NSCLC[*], RCC[*]	Genentech
BEC2	Mitumomab	Mouse	Anti-idiotypic, ganglioside GD3 mimic	Small cell lung carcinoma	ImClone Systems, Merck KG
Zamyl	HuM195	Humanised	CD33	AML[*]	Protein Design Labs
Lympho CIDE	Epratuzumab	Humanised	CD22	NHL[*]	ImmunoMedics, Amgen
Oncolym	^{131}I-LymI	Mouse	HLA-DR 10	NHL[*]	Peregrine
OvaRex	Oregovamab	Mouse	Tumor Ag CA125	Ovarian cancers	AltaRex
Theragyn, HMFG1	Pemtumomab	Mouse	MUC-1	Ovarian cancers	Antisoma
Cotara	^{131}I-chTNT-1/B	Chimeric	DNA-associated antigens	Glioma	Peregrine
MDX-210		Partially humanised	bispecific HER2Neu/ CD64	Breast, ovarian,prostate cancers, RCC[*]	Medarex, IDM

[*]NHL: non-Hodgkin's lymphoma; CRC : colorectal cancer; NSCLC: non-small-cell lung cancer ; RCC: renal cell carcinoma; AML: acute myelogenous leukaemia

[+]Bexxar is under advanced FDA acceptation procedure (due July 2003)

[§] Marketers/Corporate sponsors

Antibodies have been approved to treat cancer diseases (six mAbs), inflammatory diseases (three mAbs), one infectious disease (one mAb), one cardio-vascular disease (one mAb), and to prevent graft rejection (three mAbs). The next coming years will see a broader use of mAbs in various pathologies where efficient drugs are not available. Table 12.2 summarises the monoclonal antibodies that are currently tested in Phase III clinical trials for cancer treatment.

The exciting power of mAbs to fight complex diseases is already highlighted by monoclonal antibodies such as anti-Tumor Necrosis Factor α (TNFα) which exhibit a remarkable efficacy in rheumatoid arthritis and Crohn's disease. Such antibodies demonstrate that it is possible to identify molecules playing a major role in multifactorial diseases whose physiopathology is still a matter of controversy.

However, it should be pointed out that the targeting of cytokines with pleiotropic effects such as TNFα may also lead to the appearance of unexpected severe side effects. The treatment of patients with anti-TNFα antibodies has led to the emergence of tuberculosis cases. More recently, it has been suggested that all three anti-TNFα antibodies on the market may be also associated with a higher incidence of non-Hodgkin's lymphoma among patients treated for Crohn's disease and rheumatoid arthritis. Thus, the side effects of therapeutic monoclonal antibodies infused to large groups of patients once these mAbs have received marketing approval should be carefully monitored, particularly when it is known that the targeted molecules exhibit opposite biological activities such as pro-inflammatory *and* anti-infectious or anti-tumour activities.

The oncology field is likely to be a field which will largely benefit from the use of therapeutic mAbs, either as adjuvants or as a first line therapy in early stages of tumour progression. However, other disorders where few drugs with a long-term efficacy are available so far, if any, should also benefit from the development of new monoclonal antibodies or from new indications of currently marketed antibodies. Therapeutic monoclonal antibodies directed against B cells illustrate this latter trend. The efficacy of anti-CD20 antibodies, which received approval for Non-Hodgkin's lymphoma, is currently explored in other B cell related disorders, both in oncology and in auto-immune diseases where unwanted pathological auto-antibodies are produced. As already pointed out for anti-TNFα antibodies, the clinical use of antibodies in inflammatory-related disorders, although promising as few therapies with a long-term efficacy are available, should be explored with care. The pleiotropic activities of cytokines and chemokines make the use of such antibodies a difficult task if one wants to avoid severe side-effects. If the mechanisms of these side effects are elucidated, it may be possible to engineer these properties out and generate more specific reagents. New strategies for *in vivo* delivery (route, doses, schedule...) may also help to control side effects. However, a case-by-case approach could be necessary, which may render difficult the use of such monoclonal antibodies at a large scale with an acceptable cost for health care systems.

Different monoclonal antibodies are currently being tested in Phase III trials, in inflammatory, auto-immune and immune-related neuro-degenerative diseases (Table 12.3).

Table 12.3. Summary of mAbs in Phase III clinical trials (inflammatory, allergic, auto-immune related diseases)

Antibody	Name	Origin	Molecular target	Indication	Company[§]
Xolair	Omalizumab	Humanised	IgE	Allergic asthma	Genentech
Antegren	Natalizumab	Humanised	Integrin α4	Crohn's disease, multiple sclerosis, inflammatory diseases	Elan-Biogen
Raptiva[+]	Efalizumab	Humanised	CD11a	Psoriasis, RA[*]	Genentech, XOMA, Serono
Humicade	CDP571	Humanised	TNFα	RA[*], Crohn's disease	Celltech, Pharmacia
HuMax-CD4		Human	CD4	RA[*]	GenMab
Segard	Afelimomab	Mouse	TNFα	Sepsis	Abbott Laboratories

[*]RA : Rheumatoid Arthritis
[§]Marketers/Corporate sponsors
[+]FDA Biological Licence Application accepted on March 2003

Similarly, although only one anti-infectious antibody is currently marketed (Table 12.1), one can expect that a growing number of monoclonal antibodies directed against infectious agents or pathogen-derived toxins will be tested in Phase II and Phase III trials in the next coming years. It is likely that the use of antibodies in infectious diseases will contribute to the development of new regulatory approaches for antibody approval as discussed below in the Conclusions section.

Monoclonal antibodies directed against new targets are currently raised at a high rate with the help of proteomics and genomics approaches. As more and more antibodies enter the product pipelines, biotech companies as well as big pharmaceutical companies will face the difficult question of production in terms of both scale and cost. On the one hand, a better affinity of the antibodies infused to patients could help reducing the amount of antibodies necessary to achieve a similar or a better clinical result. In addition, the optimisation of the antibody effector functions is currently explored by a number of companies and academic groups. However, it is still unclear whether a gain in affinity – a technical field that has reached full maturity- and/or in the efficacy of effector functions will translate into a much lower amount of the antibody injected and/or a better efficacy. On the other hand, companies are looking into alternative techniques of antibody production, ranging from the use of new organisms for *in vitro* production to the production of human antibodies into transgenic animals or plants.

2. OPTIMISATION OF FCγ FUNCTIONS OF THERAPEUTIC ANTIBODIES

One exciting approach to optimise antibody functions and, hence, to possibly reduce the amount of antibody needed for injection, is to engineer their affinity. Many methods have been described that make it possible to obtain antibodies with sub-nanomolar affinities (Hawkins *et al.*, 1992; Vaughan *et al.*, 1996; Hoogenboom, 1997). It has been largely documented and will not be discussed in the present chapter. Monoclonal antibodies may act directly on their cellular targets by inducing neutralisation of biological functions of the targeted molecules, by inhibiting cell proliferation or by inducing programmed cell death. Thus, one can expect that a better affinity of antibodies will lead to a better capacity to exert these biological effects, although it has not been yet definitely proved *in vivo*.

Moreover, antibodies elicit effector functions following interactions between their Fc region and different types of receptors (FcR), as well as with C1q, the first molecule to be recruited during the activation of the classical complement pathway. The majority of therapeutic monoclonal antibodies are IgG antibodies (mostly IgG1, and in some cases, IgG4). Thus, they can interact with FcγR both *in vitro* and *in vivo*. Among FcγR, the activating FcγRs induce antibody-dependent cell cytotoxicity (ADCC), endocytosis of immune complexes followed by antigen presentation, phagocytosis, and/or release of cytokines, chemokines and pro-inflammatory mediators. The inhibitory FcγR regulates immune responses by inhibiting the activation of B lymphocytes, monocytes, mast cells and basophils, induced through activating receptors. Studies with K.O. mice support the critical role of the different types of FcγR in the functional effects of monoclonal antibodies.

Human FcγR are divided into three classes: FcγRI (CD64), FcγRII (CD32) and FcγRIII (CD16). FcγRI is a high affinity receptor and binds both monomeric IgG and immune complexes, whereas FcγRII and FcγRIII exhibit a lower affinity and bind immune complexes (Hulett and Hogarth, 1994). However, FcγRIII exhibit an intermediate affinity (Maenaka *et al.*, 2001) and is likely to bind at least some monomeric glycoforms of human IgG1.

The FcγRIII family includes two members: FcγRIIIA, which is a transmembrane isoform weakly expressed on macrophages, a subpopulation of monocytes, some γδ T cells but strongly expressed on NK cells. FcγRIIIB has a GPI (glycosyl-phosphatidyl-inositol) anchor and is expressed on neutrophils. Induction of effector functions through FcγRI and FcγRIIIA requires the presence of an additional subunit, the γ-chain, responsible for signal transduction through ITAM (Immunoreceptor Tyrosine-based Activation Motif) motifs (Amigorena *et al.,*1992; Daëron *et al.*, 1995). Gamma-chain K.O. mice show a lack of expression of FcγRI and FcγRIII, exhibit impaired ADCC, including a loss of NK cell-mediated ADCC, as well as an impaired phagocytosis of IgG1-opsonized particles. Furthermore, these mice fail to demonstrate protective tumour immunity in models of passive and active immunisation against a relevant tumour differentiation antigen, gp75, expressed on melanoma (Clynes *et al.*, 1998). In wild-type mice, passive immunisation with a monoclonal antibody against gp75 prevents the development of lung metastases, whereas this protective response is completely abolished in these FcRγ-deficient mice.

The FcγRII family includes five types of receptors (FcγRIIA1, A2, B1, B2, B3, and C). Among these receptors, FcγRIIA1, an activating receptor expressed on monocytes, macrophages, neutrophils and platelets, is characterised by the presence of an ITAM motif in the intracytoplasmic domain. The inhibitory receptors FcγRIIB1 and FcγRIIB2, expressed on B cells, basophils, mast cells, monocytes, macrophages and dendritic cells, have an intracytoplasmic ITIM (Immunoreceptor Tyrosine-based Inhibition Motif) motif (Amigorena *et al.*, 1992; Daëron *et al*, 1995). FcγRIIB-deficient mice show a functional defect in the expression of FcγRIIB1 on B cells and FcγRIIB2 on macrophages and mast cells. These mice display elevated immunoglobulin levels to immunisation with thymus-dependent or thymus-independent antigens, and show an important cutaneous anaphylaxis (Takaï *et al.*, 1996). Studies with FcγR[-/-] mice have revealed some mechanisms of action *in vivo* of two widely used therapeutic monoclonal antibodies: Herceptin and Rituxan are two cytotoxic monoclonal antibodies against tumours (Table 12.1), and engage both activating (FcγRIII) and inhibitory (FcγRIIB) receptors on myeloid cells. In these studies, FcγRIIB-deficient mice showed more ADCC than wild-type mice, whereas mice deficient in FcγRIII were unable to stop the tumour growth even in presence of therapeutic monoclonal antibodies (Clynes *et al.*, 2000). Other studies about the role of FcγR on dendritic cells (DCs) indicated that FcγRIIB[-/-] DCs have an enhanced ability to prime antigen-specific CD8[+] T lymphocytes *in vivo*, inducing an effective antigen-specific anti-tumour immune response (Kalergis and Ravetch, 2002). These studies show the potent role of FcγRIIB in the negative regulation of monoclonal antibodies effector functions. Thus, the therapeutic efficacy of monoclonal antibodies may depend on the activation or on the negative regulation of immune effector functions rather than on intrinsic events triggered by their binding to the targeted molecules. In such cases, it may be of particular interest to optimise the interactions between the Fc region and FcγR. Cytotoxic monoclonal antibodies with enhanced engagement of activating FcγR and reduced binding to inhibitory FcγR could elicit increased anti-tumour or anti-viral efficacy. Furthermore, monoclonal antibodies that recruit and activate preferentially inhibitory FcγR could be used in the treatment of autoimmune diseases.

Engineering the Fc region of IgG monoclonal antibodies to improve effector functions is a major goal of numerous studies currently developed. It has been shown that a number of amino-acid residues present in the Fc region of human IgG1 are critical for FcγR interaction, (Shields *et al.*, 2001). A common set of IgG1 residues is involved in binding to all FcγR since their mutation reduces binding to all FcγR. Alteration of some other residues improves the binding to a specific FcγR without affecting binding to the other receptors. Alternatively, mutations of several positions improve the binding to one type of FcγR and reduce the binding to another type. These experiments have also indicated that the variants with enhanced binding to FcγRIIIA exhibit enhanced ADCC *in vitro*.

A different approach to increase the biological activity of IgG is to engineer the glycosylation pattern of the Fc region. An IgG molecule contains, on each heavy chain, an oligosaccharide covalently attached at the conserved Asn297 of the CH2 domain in the Fc region. The IgG glycosylation is essential for effector functions (complement recruitment and FcγR engagement). Some studies showed that the oligosaccharide is likely to stabilise the conformation of Fcγ binding site on Fc (Radaev *et al.*, 2001). It has been hypothesised that deglycosylation causes a conformational change in the relative orientation of the two CH2 domains and that the Fc transition from an open to a closed conformation could prevent FcγR binding (Radaev and Sun, 2001).

The oligosaccharide found in the Fc region of serum IgGs is a biantennary complex [Asn 297-GlcNac-GlcNac-Mannose-(Mannose-GlcNac)$_2$], where GlcNac is N-acetylglucosamine. Variations of IgG glycosylation patterns include attachment of terminal sialic acid, a third GlcNAc arm (bisecting GlNac), terminal galactosylation and core fucosylation. Oligosaccharides can contain zero (G0), one (G1), or two (G2) galactose (Fig. 12.1).

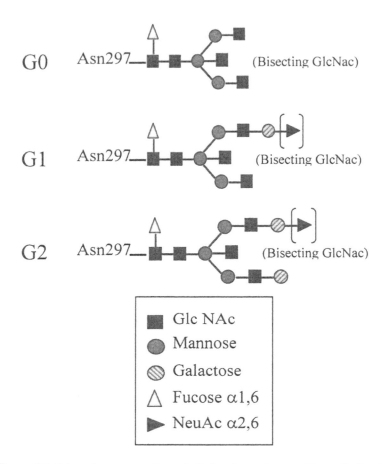

Figure 12.1. Schematic representation of IgG glycoforms. Sugar residues of IgG carbohydrate include N-acetylglucosamine (GlcNac), mannose, galactose, fucose, and sialic acid (NeuAc). The variations in IgG glycoforms depend on the attachment of galactose, NeuAc residues and of bisecting GlcNac to the core GlcNac$_2$Man$_3$GlcNac. Oligosaccharides may contain zero (G0), one (G1) or two (G2) galactose residues. Variations in the number of the different carbohydrate residues have an effect on IgG effector functions.

The pattern of glycosylation may depend on the structural properties of IgG subcomponents, in particular CH2 and CH3 domains (Lund *et al.,* 2000). However, the cell lines used to produce recombinant IgG may also influence the synthesis of oligosaccharide chains. The cells lines (essentially derived from mouse and hamster cell lines) used for recombinant monoclonal antibodies production normally attach oligosaccharides in a manner very similar to that found for serum IgGs. However, current studies try to engineer these cell lines to produce recombinant IgG with well-defined pattern of glycosylation. Thus, Chinese hamster ovary cell lines (CHO) have been engineered to express high levels of human beta 1,4-galactosyltransferase (GT) and/or alpha 2,3-sialyltransferase (ST). The structure of IgG oligosaccharides produced in these cells shows a greater homogeneity as compared to control cell lines. Overexpression of GT reduces the rate of terminal GlcNAc, whereas overexpression of ST increases sialylation of oligosaccharides (Weikert *et al.*, 1999).

IgG carbohydrate influences the complement activation initiated by IgG1 binding to C1q. First, in autoimmune diseases such as rheumatoid arthritis (RA) or systemic lupus erythematosus (SLE), there is a decrease in the content of galactose residues in oligosaccharide chains of serum IgG (Groenink *et al.*, 1996; Tsuchiya *et al.*, 1989). These degalactosylated isoforms could interact with mannose binding protein (MBP), a serum protein structurally similar to C1q. This unconventional interaction of IgG could contribute to the chronic inflammation associated with RA (Malhotra *et al.*, 1995). However, the contribution of agalactosylated IgG to the phenotype of these autoimmune diseases remains a matter of controversy. Second, studies showed that a high mannose isoform of IgG cannot bind C1q, and thus activate complement. They also indicated a slightly reduced affinity for FcγRI (Wright and Morrison, 1998).

Recently, it has been shown that engineering IgG glycoforms may lead to an optimised FcγRIII-dependent ADCC, a mechanism highly sensitive to variations of the oligosaccharide structure. Whereas the terminal sialic acid seems to have no effect on ADCC (Boyd *et al.*, 1995), the impact of galactosylation of IgG oligosaccharide on ADCC is controversial. Removal of the majority of the galactose residues from a humanised monoclonal antibody IgG1 (CAMPATH-1H) reduces complement lysis activity, but has no effect on ADCC (Boyd *et al.*, 1995). However, studies have shown that a highly galactosylated form of BRAD-3, a human anti-RhD monoclonal IgG, is more active in ADCC assays than the agalactosyl form (Kumpel *et al.*, 1994). Moreover, BRAD-5, another anti-RhD monoclonal antibody, elicites a reduced ADCC through FcγRIII after treatment with beta-galactosidase (Kumpel *et al.*, 1995). Several studies have focused on the role of bisecting GlcNAc in binding to FcγRIII and ADCC. The glycosylation pattern of a chimeric IgG1 anti-neuroblastoma antibody has been engineered in CHO cells transfected with beta 1,4-N-acetylglucosaminyltransferase III (GnTIII) (Umana *et al.*, 1999). This enzyme catalyses the addition of bisecting GlcNAc residue to the N-linked oligosaccharide. IgG variants produced in this cell line exhibit an increased ADCC. Moreover, expression of GnTIII in a recombinant anti-CD20 CHO production cell line increases the rate of bisecting GlcNAc anti-CD20 glycoforms. These antibodies elicit an increased binding to FcγRIII and a greater ADCC activity (Davies *et al.*,

2001). However the contribution of bisecting GlcNAc on effector functions is a matter of controversy. An anti-human interleukin 5 receptor (hIL-5R) humanised IgG1 and an anti-CD20 chimeric IgG1 have been produced in rat hybridoma YB2/0 cell lines (Shinkawa *et al.*, 2003). YB2/0 cells express a lower level of alpha 1,6-fucosyltransferase, and YB2/0-produced IgG1 have lower fucosylated oligosaccharide than CHO-produced IgG1. These studies have shown that non-fucosylated oligosaccharides play a more critical role in enhancing ADCC than bisecting GlcNAc oligosaccharides. It confirms previous experiments performed by Shields *et al.* (2002) who studied the effects of low-fucosylated oligosaccharides on antibody effector functions. In these studies, the fucose deficiency of IgG1 had no effect on C1q binding but provoked an increased binding to human FcγRIIIA and allowed a higher ADCC activity. However, the combined effect of each sugar residues on FcγR binding and ADCC has not been yet analysed. Moreover, all these results do not take in account FcγR polymorphisms (Hulett and Hogarth, 1994), which seem to be directly involved in the efficacy of therapeutic antibodies, as recently shown for the anti-CD20 antibody Rituximab (Cartron *et al.*, 2002).

3.   CONCLUSIONS

Up to now, fourteen monoclonal antibodies are on the market and generate revenues of about five billions Euros per year. Over the last decade, therapeutic antibodies have moved to the forefront of protein drug development and the coming years will see a new wave of recombinant antibodies in a number of indications where efficient drugs are not available. One can also expect that antibody-derived molecules, such as single chain Fv (scFv) antibody fragments, minibodies, single antibody domains, short protein scaffolds grafted with hypervariable regions of antibodies, will find a place of choice in the therapeutic arsenal. These molecules offer the advantage of being produced more easily in bacterial systems at lower costs, and do not show the practical limitations of the pharmacology of intact antibodies. Notably, small antibody fragments demonstrated rapid and high tumour uptake, whereas only limited quantities of intact antibodies are delivered to tumours, with a relatively poor diffusion from the vasculature into and through the tumour. Antibodies chemically coupled to radionucleides or antibiotics, or fused to toxins, cytokines, chemokines or growth factors are also coming of age as therapeutics. It is interesting to note that two out of the fourteen antibodies that received approval are chemically coupled molecules, either to a radionucleide (^{90}Y) or to a drug (Ozogamicin) (Table 1).

However, therapeutic antibodies still face important challenges. A careful examination of the clinical responses obtained with many of the currently marketed antibodies shows that only a low percentage of patients exhibits long-lasting complete responses to treatments, particularly in cancer treatments. Furthermore, severe side effects such as the appearance of tuberculosis or lymphomas, the worsening of heart failure, an increased cardio-cytotoxicity when combined with anthracyclin-based chemotherapy, have been described for some marketed antibodies. Thus, there is still a need to enhance the efficacy of therapeutic antibodies, while lowering the side effects that are observed for some of them. It may be achieved by further molecular engineering that will improve the affinity and/or the avidity of the antibodies for the targeted molecule. In parallel, molecular modeling of the Fc region will help to recruit either the activating or the inhibitory FcγRs depending of the disorder being targeted. Our detailed knowledge on the structure and functions of antibodies as well as the formidable possibilities offered by current molecular and cellular engineering techniques should make it possible to achieve these goals in a near future. Also, parameters such as antibody doses, routes and schemes of infusion are likely to be important parameters to obtain long lasting complete responses. Efforts to ameliorate the pharmacokinetics and the bio-availability of the antibodies are also crucial. Ultimately, one can think that a better knowledge of the physiopathology of the disorder that is being targeted should help to design *à la carte* more efficient antibodies.

Progress concerning all these aspects should permit to significantly lower the amount of antibodies required to treat patients. Better clinical outcomes with lower amounts of antibodies should lead to a decrease of the direct cost of antibody treatment as well as to important savings on the cost of the global health care *per* patient. The cost of therapeutic antibodies should be also decreased by the development of new production methods either *in vitro* (fungi, yeast, bacteria, insect cells) or in transgenic plants (corn, soybean, tobacco) or animals (cows, goats, rabbits, chicken). The problems encountered when an optimised glycosylation is needed should be solved by a fine tuning of the glycosylation process, thanks to the power of molecular engineering adapted to the manipulation of glycosylation-related enzymes.

An important and well-known problem encountered during tumour treatment is the loss or the down-modulation of the epitope recognised by the monoclonal antibody. It is also observed with various pathogens including viruses and parasites. This phenomenon is likely to hamper the clinical outcome in many cases. A strategy to overcome this problem is to use several monoclonal antibodies that recognise different epitopes or molecules on the tumour cells or on the infected cells. It has been also shown that a mixture of several antibodies is more efficient than a single antibody to neutralise dangerous toxins that can be used as weapons of mass destruction. Thus, the use of a mixture of human monoclonal antibodies, eventually with different effector functions, could be more efficient than the use of a single antibody in the treatment of certain cancers and of some infectious diseases. Although the actual cost of development and production of therapeutic monoclonal antibodies may render this approach unrealistic, one can think that this question will be opened for discussion in a near future. Progress in the antibody production and purification techniques as well as changes in the current rules for antibody approval should allow to envision the simultaneous use of several monoclonal antibodies. Alternatively, the capacity of producing human antibodies in large amount in transgenic cows (Kuroiwa *et al.*, 2002) should allow to revisit the use of ... polyclonal antibodies as therapeutics.

ACKNOWLEDGEMENTS

We would like to thank all our colleagues who participated in our work on monoclonal antibodies over the last decade. We also thank Pr. W.H. Fridman for constant support. S. Sibéril is supported by a CIFRE fellowship from the ANRT (no. 773/2001) and the Laboratoire Français du Fractionnement et des Biotechnologies (LFB, Les Ulis, France).

REFERENCES

Amigorena S., Bonnerot C., Drake J., Choquet D., Hunziker W., Guillet J.G., Webster P., Sautes C., Mellman I., and Fridman W.H., 1992, Cytoplasmic domain heterogeneity and functions of IgG Fc receptors in B-lymphocytes. *Science* **256**: 1808-1812
Banchereau, J., de Paoli, P., Valle, A., Garcia, E., and Rousset, F., 1989, Long-term human B cell lines dependent on interleukin-4 and antibody to CD40. *Science* **251**: 70-72
Borrebaeck, C.A.K., 1989, Strategy for the production of human monoclonal antibodies using *in vitro* activated B cells. *J. Immunol. Methods* **123**: 157-165
Boyd, P.N., Lines, A.C., and Patel, A.K., 1995, The effect of the removal of sialic acid, galactose and total carbohydrate on the functional activity of Campath-1H. *Mol. Immunol.* **32**: 1311-1318
Cartron, G., Dacheux, L., Salles, G., Solal-Celigny, P., Bardos, P., Colombs, P., and Watier, H., 2002, Therapeutic activity of humanized anti-CD20 monoclonal antibody and polymorphism in IgG Fc receptor FcgammaRIIIa gene. *Blood* **99**: 754-758
Clynes, R., Takechi, Y., Moroi, Y., Houghton, A., and Ravetch, J.V., 1998, Fc receptors are required in passive and active immunity to melanoma. *Proc. Natl. Acad. Sci. USA* **95**: 652-656
Clynes, R.A., Towers, T.L., Presta, L.G., and Ravetch, J.V., 2000, Inhibitory Fc receptors modulate *in vivo* cytoxicity against tumor targets. *Nature Med.* **6**: 443-446

Co, M.S. and Queen, C., 1991, Humanized antibodies for therapy. *Nature* 351: 501-502

Daëron, M., Latour, S., Malbec, O., Espinosa, E., Pina, P., Pasmans, S., and Fridman, W.H., 1995, The same tyrosine-based inhibition motif, in the intracytoplasmic domain of FcγRIIB, regulates negatively BCR-, TCR-, and FcR-dependent cell activation. *Immunity* 3: 635-646

Davies, J., Jiang, L., Pan, L.Z., LaBarre, M.J., Anderson, D., and Reff, M., 2001, Expression of GnTIII in a recombinant anti-CD20 CHO production cell line: expression of antibodies with altered glycoforms leads to an increase in ADCC through higher affinity for Fcgamma RIII. *Biotechnol. Bioeng.* 74: 188-294

Green, L.L., Hardy, M.C., Maynard-Currie, C.E., Tsuda, H., Louie, D.M., Mendez, M.J., Abderrahim, H., Noguchi, M., Smith, D.H., Zeng, Y., et al., 1994, Antigen-specific human monoclonal antibodies from mice engineered with human Ig heavy and light chain YACs. *Nature Genet.* 7:13-21

Groenink, J., Spijker, J., van den Herik-Oudijk, I.E., Boeije, L., Rook, G., Aarden, L., Smeenk, R., van de Winkel, J.G., and van den Broek, M.F., 1996, On the interaction between agalactosyl IgG and Fc gamma receptors. *Eur. J. Immunol.* 26: 1404-1407

Hawkins, R.E., Russell, S.J., and Winter, G., 1992, Selection of phage antibodies by binding affinity: mimicking affinity maturation. *J. Mol. Biol.* 226: 889-896

Hoogenboom, H.R., 1997, Designing and optimizing library selection strategies for generating high-affinity antibodies. *Trends Biotechnol.* 15: 62-70

Hulett, M.D., and Hogarth, P.M., 1994, Molecular basis of Fc receptor function. *Adv. Immunol.* 57: 1-127

Huse, W.D., Sastry, L., Iverson, S.A., Kang, A.S., Alting, M.M., Burton, D.R., Benkovic, S.J., and Lerner, R.A., 1989, Generation of a large combinatorial library of the immunoglobulin repertoire in phage lambda. *Science* 246: 1275-1281

Kalergis, A.M., and Ravetch, J.V., 2002, Inducing tumor immunity through the selective engagement of activating Fcgamma receptors on dendritic cells. *J. Exp. Med.* 195: 1653-1659

Köhler, G. and Milstein, C., 1975, Continuous cultures of fused cells secreting antibody of predefined specificity. *Nature* 256: 495-497

Kumpel, B.M., Rademacher, T.W., Rook, G.A., Williams, P.J., and Wilson, I.B., 1994, Galactosylation of human IgG monoclonal anti-D produced by EBV-transformed B-lymphoblastoid cell lines is dependent on culture method and affects Fc receptor-mediated functional activity. *Hum. Antibodies Hybridomas.* 5: 143-151

Kumpel, B.M., Wang, Y., Griffiths, H.L., Hadley, A.G., and Rook, G.A., 1995, The biological activity of human monoclonal IgG anti-D is reduced by beta-galactosidase treatment. *Hum. Antibodies Hybridomas.* 6: 82-88

Kuroiwa, Y., Kasinathan, P., Choi, Y.J., Naeem, R., Tomizuka, K., Sullivan, E.J., Knott, J.G., Duteau, A., Goldsby, R.A., Osborne, B .A., Ishida, I., and Robl, J.M., (2002) Cloned transchromosomic calves producing human immunoglobulin. *Nature Biotechnol.* 20: 889-894

Lonberg, N., Taylor, L.D., Harding, F.A., Trounstine, M., Higgins, K.M., Schramm, S.R., Kuo, C.C., Mashayekh, R., Wymore, K., McCabe, J.G., et al. 1994, Antigen-specific human antibodies from mice comprising four distinct genetic modifications. *Nature* 368: 856-859

Lund, J., Takahashi, N., Popplewell, A., Goodall, M., Pound, J.D., Tyler, R., King, D.J., and Jefferis, R., 2000, Expression and characterization of truncated forms of humanized L243 IgG1. Architectural features can influence synthesis of its oligosaccharide chains and affect superoxide production triggered through human Fcgamma receptor I. *Eur. J. Biochem.* 267: 7246-7257

Maenaka, K., van der Merwe, P.A., Stuart, D.I., Jones, E.Y., and Sondermann, P., 2001, The human low affinity Fcgamma receptors IIa, IIb, and III bind IgG with fast kinetics and distinct thermodynamic properties. *J. Biol. Chem.* **276**: 44898-44904

Malhotra, R., Wormald, M.R., Rudd, P.M., Fischer, P.B., Dwek, R.A., and Sim, R.B., 1995, Glycosylation changes of IgG associated with rheumatoid arthritis can activate complement via the mannose-binding protein. *Nature Med.* **1**: 237-243

McCafferty, J., Griffiths, A.D., Winter, G., and Chiswell, D.J., 1990, Phage antibodies: filamentous phage displaying antibody variable domains. *Nature* **348**: 552-554

Morrison, S.L., Johnson, M.J., Herzenberg, L.A., and Oi, V.T., 1984, Chimeric human antibody molecules : mouse antigen-binding domains with human constant region domains. *Proc Natl Acad Sci USA* **81**: 6851-6855

Olsson, L. and Kaplan, H.S., 1980, Human-human hybridomas producing monoclonal antibodies of predefined antigenic specificity. *Proc. Natl. Acad. Sci. USA* **77**: 5429-5431

Queen, C., Schneider, W.P., Selick, H.E., Payne, P.W., Landolfi, N.F., Duncan, J.F., Avdalovic, N.M., Levitt, M., Junghans, R.P., and Waldmann, T.A., 1989, A humanized antibody that binds to the interleukin 2 receptor. *Proc. Natl. Acad. Sci. USA* **86**: 10029-10035

Radaev, S., Motyka, S., Fridman, W.H., Sautes-Fridman, C., and Sun, P.D., 2001, The structure of a human type III Fcgamma receptor in complex with Fc. *J. Biol. Chem.* **276**: 16469-16477

Radaev, S., and Sun, P.D., 2001, Recognition of IgG by Fcgamma receptor. The role of Fc glycosylation and the binding of peptide inhibitors. *J. Biol. Chem.* **276**: 16478-16483

Shields, R.L., Lai, J., Keck, R., O'Connell, L.Y., Hong, K., Meng, Y.G., Weikert, S.H., and Presta, L.G., 2002, Lack of fucose on human IgG1 N-linked oligosaccharide improves binding to human Fcgamma RIII and antibody-dependent cellular toxicity. *J. Biol. Chem.* **277**: 26733-26740

Shields, R.L., Namenuk, A.K., Hong, K., Meng, Y.G., Rae, J., Briggs, J., Xie, D., Lai, J., Stadlen, A., Li, B., Fox, J.A., and Presta, L.G., 2001, High resolution mapping of the binding site on human IgG1 for Fcgamma RI, Fcgamma RII, Fcgamma RIII, and FcRn and design of IgG1 variants with improved binding to the Fcgamma R. *J. Biol. Chem.* **276**: 6591-6604

Shinkawa, T., Nakamura, K., Yamane, N., Shoji-Hosaka, E., Kanda, Y., Sakurada, M., Uchida, K., Anazawa, H., Satoh, M., Yamasaki, M., Hanai, N., and Shitara, K., 2003, The absence of fucose but not the presence of galactose or bisecting N-acetylglucosamine of human IgG1 complex-type oligosaccharides shows the critical role of enhancing antibody-dependent cellular cytotoxicity. *J. Biol. Chem.* **278**: 3466-3473

Smith, G.P., 1985, Filamentous fusion phage: novel expression vectors that display cloned antigens on the virion surface. *Science* **228**: 1315-1317

Steinitz, M., Klein, G., Koskimies, S., and Makela, O., 1977, EB virus induced B lymphocyte cell lines producing specific antibodies. *Nature* **269**: 420-422

Takai, T., Ono, M., Hikida, M., Ohmori, H., and Ravetch, J.V., 1996, Augmented humoral and anaphylactic responses in Fc gamma RII-deficient mice. *Nature* **379**: 346-349

Takeda, S.I., Naito, T., Hama, K., Noma, T., and Honjo, T., 1985, Construction of chimæric processed immunoglobulin genes containing mouse variable and human constant region sequences. *Nature* **314**: 452-454

Tomizuka, K., Shinohara, T., Yoshida, H., Uejima, H., Ohguma, A., Tanaka, S., Sato, K., Oshimura, M., and Ishida, I., 2000, Double trans-chromosomic mice: maintenance of two individual human chromosome fragments containing Ig heavy and kappa loci and expression of fully human antibodies. *Proc. Natl. Acad. Sci. USA* **97**: 722-727

Tsuchiya, N., Endo, T., Matsuta, K., Yoshinoya, S., Aikawa, T., Kosuge, E., Takeuchi, F., Miyamoto T., and Kobata A., 1989, Effects of galactose depletion from oligosaccharide chains on immunological activities of human IgG. *J. Rheumatol.* **16**: 285-290

Umana, P., Jean-Mairet, J., Moudry, R., Amstutz, H., and Bailey J.E., 1999, Engineered glycoforms of an antineuroblastoma IgG1 with optimized antibody-dependent cellular cytotoxic activity. *Nat. Biotechnol.* **17**: 176-180

Vaughan, T.J., Williams, A.J., Pritchard, K., Osbourn, J.K., Pope, A.R., Earnshaw, J.C., McCafferty, J., Hodits, R.A., Wilton, J., and Johnson, K.S., 1996, Human antibodies with sub-nanomolar affinities isolated from a large non-immunized phage display library. *Nat. Biotechnol.* **14**:309-314

Weikert, S., Papac, D., Briggs, J., Cowfer, D., Tom, S., Gawlitzek, M., Lofgren, J., Mehta, S., Chisholm, V., Modi, N., Eppler, S., Carroll, K., Chamow, S., Peers, D., Berman, P., and Krummen, L., 1999, Engineering Chinese hamster ovary cells to maximize sialic acid content of recombinant glycoproteins. *Nat. Biotechnol.* **17**: 1116-1121

Wright, A., and Morrison S.L., 1998, Effect of C2-associated carbohydrate structure on Ig effector function: studies with chimeric mouse-human IgG1 antibodies in glycosylation mutants of Chinese hamster ovary cells. *J. Immunol.* **160**: 3393-3402

Index